ultrasonography
of the abdomen

ultrasonography of the abdomen

by N. Hassani

(with a contribution by R. Bard)

includes 215 illustrations

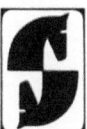

Springer-Verlag
New York Heidelberg Berlin
1976

N. Hassani, M.D.
Assistant Professor of Radiology
State University of New York at Stony Brook and
Physician in Charge, Ultrasound Division, Department of Radiology
Queens Hospital Center
87-15 165th Street
Jamaica, New York 11432

R. Bard, M.D.
Ultrasound Department
New York Medical College
1249 Fifth Avenue
New York, New York 10029

Library of Congress Cataloging in Publication Data

Hassani, Nasser, 1938-
   Ultrasonography of the abdomen.

   Bibliography: p. 119
   Includes index.
   1. Abdomen—Diseases—Diagnosis.   2. Diagnosis, Ultrasonic.   I. Title.
[DNLM: 1. Abdomen.   2. Ultrasonics—Diagnostic use. WI900 H353u]
RC944.H32   617′.55′0754   76-15316

Softcover reprint of the hardcover 1st edition 1976

ISBN-13: 978-1-4612-9871-7   e-ISBN-13: 978-1-4612-9869-4
DOI: 10.1007/978-1-4612-9869-4

foreword

by Dr. Jan. J. Smulewicz

Ultrasound imaging has reached a stage of sophistication whereby diagnostic information can be gained without discomfort to the patient and with complete absence of morbidity and mortality. The procedure is quick, safe, noninvasive and in many instances can supersede and obviate more time-consuming procedures requiring catheterization, injection of a contrast material, and radiographic imaging. In obstetrical problems the danger of ionizing radiation to the fetus is eliminated. In debilitated and very ill patients this simple and painless method becomes the procedure of choice.

Unique features of ultrasound equipment allow for pinpoint localization of lesions and direct visual guidance of percutaneous puncture techniques for aspiration and biopsy. The accuracy of ultrasound guided punctures and the absence of side effects make this modality far superior to percutaneous invasive techniques performed with other imaging systems. Renal cyst puncture and amniocentesis are but two of the procedures in which ultrasonic guidance is the method of choice.

Dr. Hassani has throughly explained and carefully explored the wide variety of examinations available with ultrasound. The large volume of material and the clear interpretation makes this book of great interest to all of the medical profession. In addition to the existing methods available for diagnostic interpretations, this method of noninvasive diagnosis should find its way into every hospital or center where good medical care is provided.

Jan J. Smulewicz, M.D.
Chairman of the Radiology Department,
Queens Hospital Center;
Professor of Radiology,
SUNY at Stony Brook

foreword

by Dr. M. Tafreshi

Diagnostic ultrasound has been extensively applied to cardiac disorders and obstetrical problems. The appearance of gray scale and real time ultrasonic scanners has now permitted sophisticated examination of the upper abdominal organs. Since this modality is noninvasive, it may be performed serially and at any given time. This sequential observation of pathophysiology in the living subject provides important data on the progression of acute and chronic diseases and their response to treatment.

The unusual accuracy of ultrasound in differentiating cystic from solid masses and its ability to localize the lesion in a three dimensional representation have rendered other diagnostic procedures unnecessary.

The standard radiologic evaluation for abdominal masses has generally included the plain x-ray film of the abdomen, intravenous urography, barium enema, gastrointestinal series, cholecystography, and radio-isotopic procedures. Invasive and time-consuming studies such as lymphangiography and arteriography have also been used, sometimes without adding further diagnostic

information. Sonography is safe and relatively
inexpensive and should be included in the
workup of a mass lesion.
Since ultrasound may give a specific diagnosis,
its application should follow the plain x-ray
film. This simple and rapid study may eliminate the need for a prolonged hospital stay
and the discomfort of further examinations.
At our institution diagnostic ultrasound has
greatly reduced the patient time spent in the
x-ray department, given the surgeon faster
and more reliable diagnostic information,
and generally speeded up the patient turnover
at the hospital. With the economic emphasis
on the reduction of the cost of medical services
and hospitalization expense, the ultrasound
department serves a vital function in facili-
tating diagnostic services.

M. Tafreshi, M.D.
Associate Director of the Radiology Department
Queens Hospital Center

preface

Major improvements in the resolution of ultrasound equipment have led to increasing application of ultrasonic sectional body imaging to all fields of medical science. The proven safety of ultrasound and its noninvasive nature has made this modality more often the diagnostic procedure of choice. These rapid and atraumatic tools are ideal for screening programs. The overwhelming acceptance of the value of cross-sectional imaging by the health sciences ensures continued development and expansion of the uses of noninvasive scanning.

The purpose of this book is to introduce the physician to the essential principles of ultrasound physics and the practical aspects of scanning procedures. Important concepts are clearly and thoroughly presented. Mathematical formulas and advanced physical principles beyond the scope of the clinician have been omitted. The text is limited to the upper abdomen in order to concentrate on each system in sufficient depth to be of value to the specialist who must be familiar with the diagnostic capabilities of atraumatic scanners in his field of interest. The methods of examination and diagnostic findings are detailed to be of use to the radiologist, the internist, and the general surgeon. The comprehensive scope serves as a general reference for both the family practitioner and the student in training.

In the sections on physical and practical applications, precise directions for examination are given and scanning pitfalls with the production of artifacts have been underscored. The evolution of scanning systems has been traced so that the potential features and limitations of each imaging unit are recognized. Representations of each type of scanning device are illustrated and their inherent advantages discussed.

Examination of each body region has been arranged so that the reader may review the pertinent regional anatomy before studying the ultrasonic presentation of normal structures. The pathology of each organ is presented as a disease spectrum and the evolution of the disorder is discussed. Correlation between sonographic findings and the histopathologic changes is emphasized. The combination of real time and gray scale scanning offers the reader a comprehensive understanding of ultrasonic pathology.

Where controversy exists, the opinions of various authorities are cited and compared with my experience. The diagnostic versatility of the various imaging systems are evaluated for each organ complex and the investigative method of choice is suggested for each disorder.

Considerable attention has been given to clinical and pathologic aspects. The practice of ultrasonic scanning requires a thorough knowledge of the diagnostic problems of medicine and surgery and their related specialties. The text is designed as a bridge between sonographic imaging and general medical and surgical principles.

acknowledgment

I wish to express my deep appreciation to Dr. Jan J. Smulewicz, and Dr. M. Tafreshi for their effort and support in establishing the ultrasound department at Queens Hospital Center. I am also very grateful to Dr. Nathaniel Finby, Professor of Radiology at Columbia University and Chairman of the Radiology Department at St. Luke's Hospital Center, and Dr. Lajos Von Micsky, Director of the Ultrasound Department at St. Luke's Hospital Center, for their dedicated guidance as my great teachers. The unstinting investigative efforts of our many colleagues in the burgeoning field of ultrasonography have greatly facilitated the evolution of this text. The support of the publishers and the collaboration of the Editorial Staff is warmly acknowledged.

N. Hassani, M.D.

introduction

From the earliest days of the application of sonic principles in medicine, there have been continuous new developments in the use of acoustical waves for diagnosis.

Historically, ultrasound was developed in World Wars I and II and was used to locate submarines. Sounding of the ocean depth was employed in 1918 to aid in shipping (47). Sonar (Sound Navigation and Ranging) used by the Navy, not only measured precisely the depth of a reflecting surface but could also track an object in motion. In 1930, ultrasound was used in industry to detect flaws in iron castings. In 1937, an ultrasonic device was designed for application to the brain (13). The first ultrasonic instrument, called the *supersonic reflectoscope*, came to the market in 1940 (17). This practical instrument, based on the pulsed-echo technique, measured distance on the principle of transmission of very short pulses of sonic energy. In 1950, sonar equipment became available in medicine.

There has been constant research with continuing new developments in this field. With the application of modern electronic equipment and rapid reporting data retrieval systems, sonography ceased to be a research project and became an important tool for the diagnosis and care of the patient.

The fundamentals of ultrasound, like any other branch of medicine, require the user to be familiar with the effects and limitations of this method. By this technique we are able to locate and measure interfaces between different organs and tissues and to cut, in cross sections through different structures. In contrast to other examinations which give indirect information, ultrasound enables us to outline the lesion directly and to investigate its relationship with neighboring structures. There is no need for the administration of any radiologic contrast, possibly harmful to the function of the impaired organ. Ultrasound, both as a screening and diagnostic modality, is a non-invasive and atraumatic procedure and is complimentary to angiography in many cases. The unique feature of ultrasound is the ability to recognize and differentiate deep body organs and lesions having similar density on conventional x-ray studies.

The information gained through ultrasound, like other imaging procedures, is optimized when coupled with the patient's clinical picture. At the present time, parenchymal lesions of the lung cannot be evaluated by ultrasound since the air-containing lung will not transmit sound waves.

contents

Foreword by Dr. Jan J. Smulewicz   v

Foreword by Dr. M. Tafreshi   vii

Preface   ix

Acknowledgment   xi

Introduction   xiii

1   principles of ultrasonography   1

CHARACTERISTICS OF ULTRASOUND   1
DISPLAY MODES   9
EQUIPMENT AND PRACTICAL ASPECTS   13
ARTIFACTS IN ULTRASONOGRAPHY   20
BIOPHYSICAL EFFECTS OF ULTRASOUND   20
GENETIC EFFECTS OF ULTRASOUND   21
PRACTICAL ASPECTS OF SONOLAPAROTOMY   21
ULTRASONIC IDENTIFICATION   23

2   hepatic sonography   29

GENERAL INTRODUCTION   29
THE LIVER   29

THE GALLBLADDER 40
THE BILIARY TREE 45

3 splenic sonography 47

GENERAL INTRODUCTION 47
THE SPLEEN 47

4 pancreatic sonography 55

GENERAL INTRODUCTION 55
THE PANCREAS 56

5 vascular sonography 72

THE ABDOMINAL AORTA 72
THE INFERIOR VENA CAVA 77

6 diaphragmatic sonography 85

GENERAL INTRODUCTION 85
THE DIAPHRAGM 85

7 sonography of ascites 89

ASCITES 89

8 sonography in planning radiation therapy 93

GENERAL INTRODUCTION 93
PATIENT CONTOUR 93
LOCALIZATION OF DEEP LESIONS 94
ORGAN EVALUATION IN RADIATION THERAPY 94
DELINEATION OF PORT MARGINS 94

9 retroperitoneal sonography 95

GENERAL INTRODUCTION 95
THE RETROPERITONEUM 95

10 renal sonography 100

GENERAL INTRODUCTION 100
THE KIDNEY 101

bibliography 119

INDEX 123

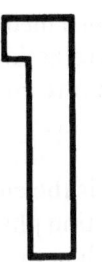

principles
of ultrasonography

CHARACTERISTICS OF ULTRASOUND

NATURE OF ULTRASONIC WAVES

Sound is a mechanical vibration of particles in a medium around an equilibrium position. Sonic waves require a medium of a molecular nature in order to propagate. The highest frequency sound audible to the human ear is 20,000 cycles per second or 20 kiloHertz (kHz). Sound waves above this frequency are described as ultrasound. Unlike electromagnetic waves, sound cannot travel across a vacuum (9).

The wavelength of audible sound in air varies from a few inches to a few feet. Ultrasonic waves are usually produced by a continuous series of contractions and relaxations of substances that have piezoelectric properties. The waves generated are carried as condensations and rarefactions in the transmitting medium. The frequency range used in diagnostic medicine is approximately one million cycles per second, with a wavelength of about 1.5 mm in water.

PIEZOELECTRIC PRINCIPLE

The piezoelectric effect is fundamental to the development of ultrasound. Piezo is derived from the Greek word *piesis,* "to press." Piezoelectric actually means "pressure electric." Quartz has piezoelectric qualities, since its size and shape change under the influence of an electric field. When an electric current is passed through quartz, the crystal expands and contracts according to the polarity of the current. Sound waves are generated as a result of these compressions and rarefactions. On the other hand, mechanical energy in the form of sound waves applied to the crystal produces an electric current. This is known as the piezoelectric principle (Fig. 1.1a and b). Several other substances are known to have piezoelectric properties, such as barium titanate, lithium sulfate, and lead zirconate (85). The titanates are the more commonly used crystal (9) for sonography.

SOUND WAVES

Sonic waves travel through a medium as alternate condensations and rarefactions. The following practical definitions are commonly used (Fig. 1.1c):

1. *Cycle.* One cycle is the entire condensation and rarefaction phase.
2. *Wavelength.* The length of one cycle is a wavelength, or, a complete condensation and rarefaction zone is a wavelength.
3. *Frequency.* The number of cycles per unit time. The frequency of sound waves is described in terms of Hertz (cycles per second).
4. *Velocity.* Velocity is the speed of sound in the medium through which sound is propagated.
   The relationship between velocity, wavelength, and frequency:

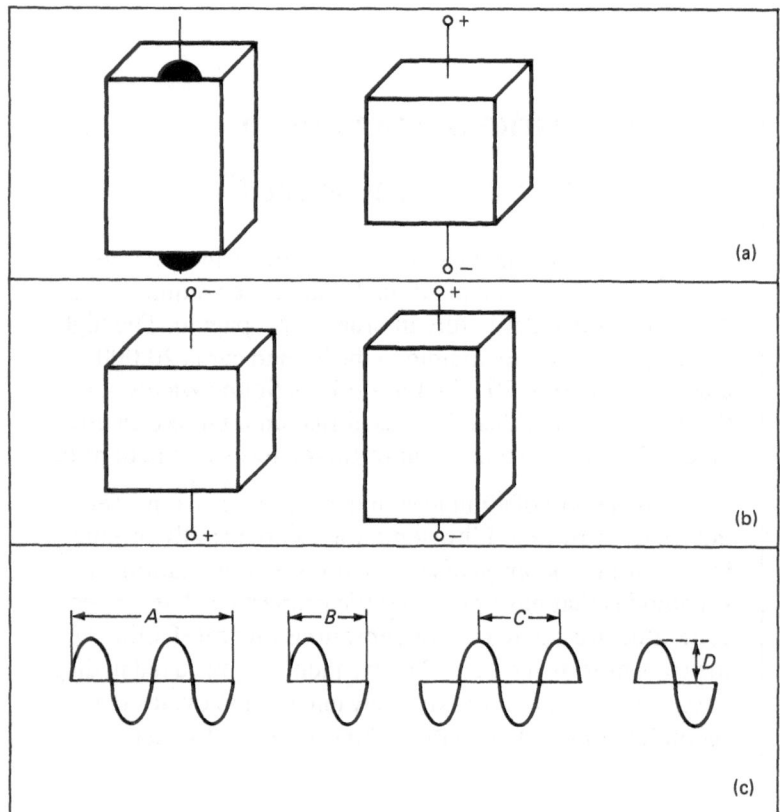

FIGURE 1.1
Piezoelectric effect. (a) Mechanical stress deforming crystal and producing current. (b) Expansion of crystal as current is applied and contraction of crystal as current polarity is reversed. (c) Wave pattern produced by alternate compressions and rarefactions. [*A*-spatial pulse length; *B*-full cycle; *C*-wavelength; *D*-amplitude.]

$$V = \lambda \times F$$
Velocity = Wavelength × Frequency

EFFECT OF MEDIUM

In any given medium the velocity of sound remains constant, but its frequency varies inversely with wavelength. The higher the frequency, the smaller the wavelength. High-frequency sound waves are more directional than low-frequency sound. However, the attenuation of high-frequency waves is greater than that of low-frequency waves, since the absorption of sound is greater at high frequency (9). In medical work, frequencies above 1 MegaHertz (MHz) are employed. At a frequency of 2 MHz, the wavelength of sound in water is approximately 0.75 mm.

Velocity depends on the density and elasticity of the medium. The elasticity of the medium is significant, since the velocity of sound changes in media of different inherent elastic properties. In a homogeneous medium, ultrasound travels in a straight line at a velocity dependent on the properties of the medium but independent of wavelength.

INTENSITY

The intensity of the ultrasound beam is a measure of the strength of its energy and is defined as power per unit area. The intensities used in commercially available medical units usually are between 1 and 40 milliWatts per square centimeter (mW/cm²). Tissue damage may occur at 4 W/cm² (24); thus, currently used intensity levels are roughly 100 to 1,000 times lower in energy than the potentially damaging level. The safety margin is much greater, since the acoustic pulse is active less than 1 percent of the scanning time.

The decibel (dB) is the practical unit for the measurement of sound intensity. The ratio of signal amplitudes must be expressed logarithmically due to the wide range of echo energies. The formula for the ratio of echo amplitude in terms of decibels is:

$$dB = 20 \log A_1/A_2$$

A_1 is the echo amplitude and A_2 the incident sound amplitude. For example, 20 dB is a factor of 10 times the intensity.

BEAM WIDTH AND ECHO PATTERN

The beam width is related to the diameter of the crystal. Ultrasonic waves transmitted from the transducer have a diverging beam width. In this path, any echo received is registered as if it were in the central beam axis (20). A target on the edge of the beam is recorded in the same way as a target in the middle.

The appearance of the displayed point is important. The echo is registered as a dot or line. The dots lie in the center of the beam and the lines are perpendicular to the beam axis of the transducer. The length of each line is proportional to the width of the beam. The apparent beam width is wider if the target is located obliquely to the incident beam. The effective beam width changes with the sensitivity of the ultrasound machine. By increasing the sensitivity of the machine, low-amplitude echoes from the edge of the beam are registered. However, the target is displayed as lines instead of dots and resolution is decreased. The geometry of the target is extremely important (Fig. 1.2a, b, and c). If the transmitted beam is stationary and at right angles to the target, the shape of the returned echo is specified by the electrical characteristics of the transducer (20). If the transmitted beam is not stationary or strikes the target obliquely, the shape of the returned echo is elongated due to a greater effective beam width with respect to the target. Thus, the echoes appear as small lines instead of dots (Fig. 1.3 a, b, and c).

ATTENUATION

When a sonic beam is passed through a medium, a decrease in the intensity of the sound, termed *attenuation,* may be expressed as a half-value layer. The half-value layer is the distance the transmitted sound must travel before its

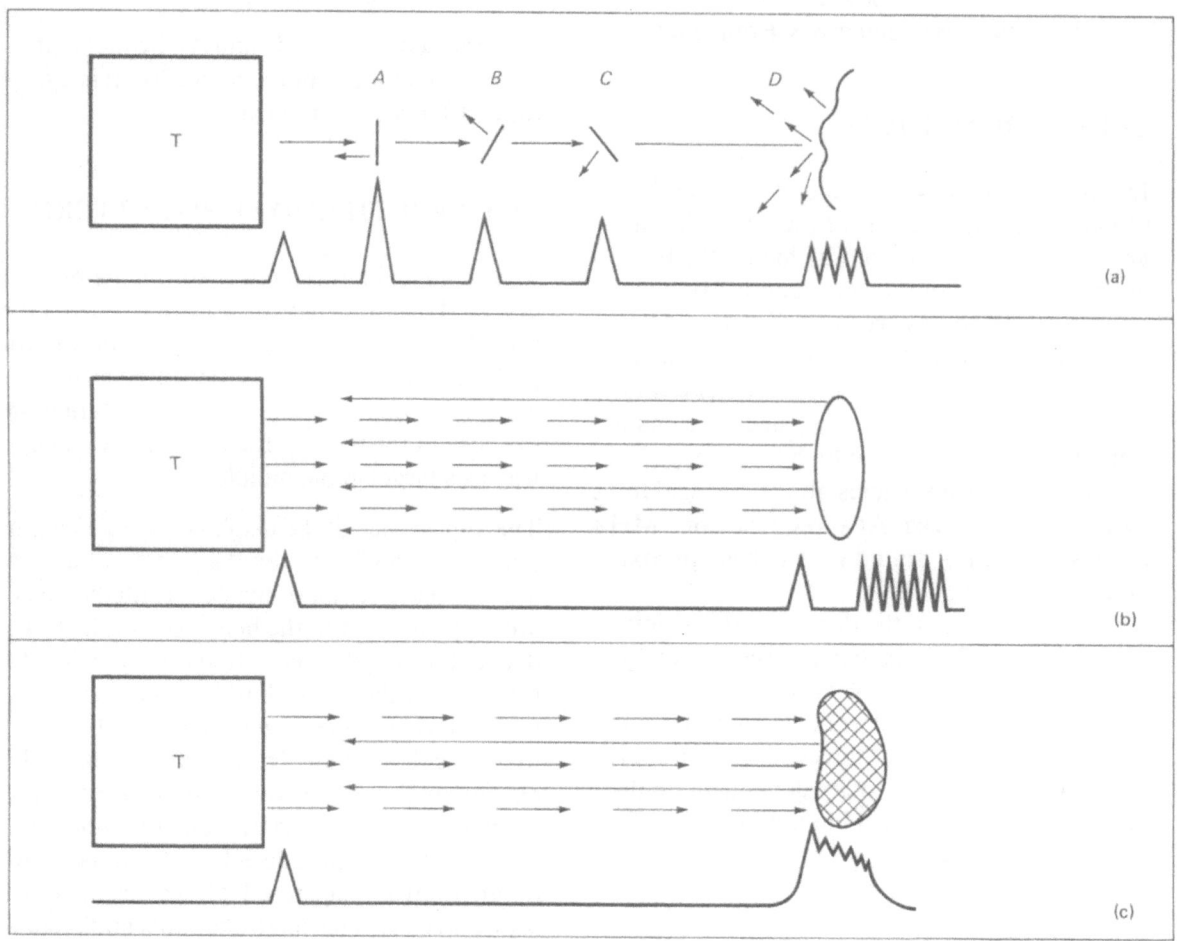

FIGURE 1.2
Reflection processes. (a) Strong echo generated by perpendicular interface (*A*). Weaker echoes due to sound reflected away from receiving transducer (*B,C*). Diffuse low level echoes from irregular reflecting interface (*D*). (b) No echoes produced as sound beam passes through homogeneous medium of cystic structure. Note high through transmission represented as multiple echoes distal to the posterior wall. (c) Echo production by solid, inhomogeneous medium. Note poor through transmission with no echoes distal to the posterior wall. [T, transducer]

initial intensity is reduced by one half. Bone has a smaller half-value layer than soft tissue (9). However, energy loss is also caused by beam divergence, scattering, and absorption of sound by tissue. The amount of sound absorbed is proportional to the depth of the tissue and the square of the frequency of sound. Attentuation of the sonic beam has many practical applications. For example, cystic and solid masses can be differentiated since cystic masses have a much greater half-value layer than solid structures. In general, soft tissue attenuation is 1dB/MHz/cm. Attenuation of bony structures is about 20 times greater than that of soft tissue. For this reason, a low-frequency transducer must be used when scanning through bony structures, such as the ribs.

ACOUSTIC IMPEDANCE

The transmissivity of the ultrasonic beam depends upon sound velocity (*V*) and the density (*D*) of the medium. The overall transmission is defined as *acoustic impedance* (*Z*). Consequently, acoustic impedance is directly related to the speed of sound in a given medium multiplied by tissue density (85).

$$Z = DV$$
$$Z = \text{Impedance}$$
$$D = \text{Density} \quad V = \text{Velocity}$$

If the interface between two media is a region of acoustic impedance mismatch, a reflection will take place proportional to the impedance differential. Each tissue has a characteristic acoustic impedance.

RESOLUTION

Resolution is the minimum distance between two point targets required to register each point as a distinct entity. The greater the resolving power, the closer the two objects may be and still be individually recognized. The resolution of any wave form is directly related to the frequency of oscillation. Higher frequency sound usually has better resolution but its intensity falls-off rapidly as it passes through a given medium (85). Lower frequency sound usually has excellent transmission but poor resolution characteristics. The frequency range between 2 and 2.5 MHz has the best balance between resolution and sound transmission for abdominal scanning. However, equipment available at the

FIGURE 1.3
Echo shape and beam path. (a) Narrow beam. Point target displayed as sharp dot. (b) Wide beam. Point target displayed as short line perpendicular to beam. (c) Narrow beam. Oblique linear target displayed as short line. [T, transducer]

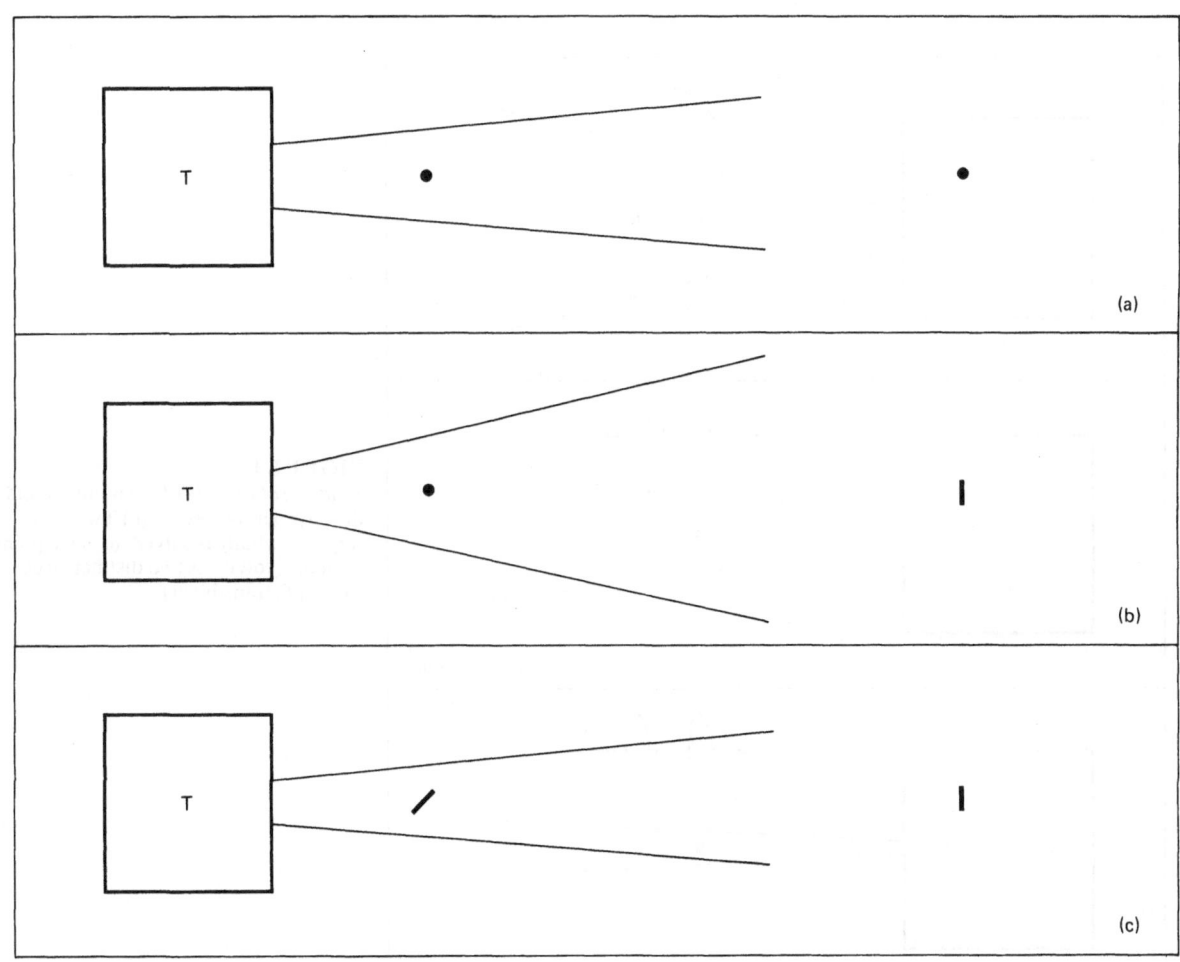

present time does not allow identification of very deep-seated abdominal structures below a certain size. Recognition of a smaller lesion depends on the overall resolution of the equipment.

In ultrasound we are concerned with axial and lateral resolution. Axial or depth resolution is the ability to distinguish two points along the beam axis (Fig. 1.4a, b, and c). The minimal resolvable distance is measured as the axial resolution and depends on wavelength, since objects separated by less than one wavelength cannot be resolved. Although the wavelengths of current transducers vary from 1.5 to 0.1 mm, the resolution of the oscilloscope, or scan converter tube, may not be sufficient to separate very closely spaced echoes. The display system must be sensitive enough to match the transducer frequency. Lateral or azimuthal resolution is the ability to distinguish two points located perpendicular to the beam axis (Fig. 1.5 a, b, and c). The minimal resolvable side-by-side distance between two objects is measured as the lateral resolution. This distance is inversely proportional to the width of the beam and depends on the diameter of the crystal, the wavelength, and the degree of beam divergence with distance.

REPETITION RATE

The rate at which bursts of ultrasonic energy are emitted is called the *repetition rate*. Most commercially available instruments emit 200–2000 repetitions per second. This high repetition rate requires extremely sensitive receivers capable of detecting a signal that has

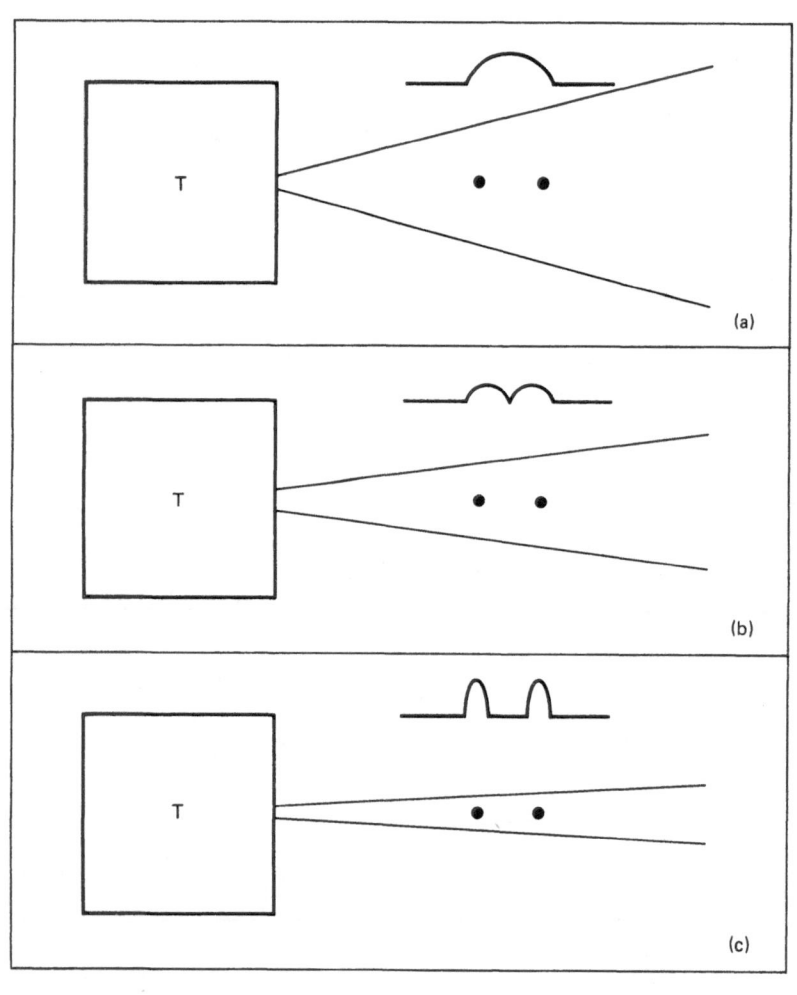

FIGURE 1.4
Axial resolution. (a) Two point targets displayed as one echo. (b) Two point targets partially resolved. (c) Two point targets resolved as two distinct structures. [T, transducer]

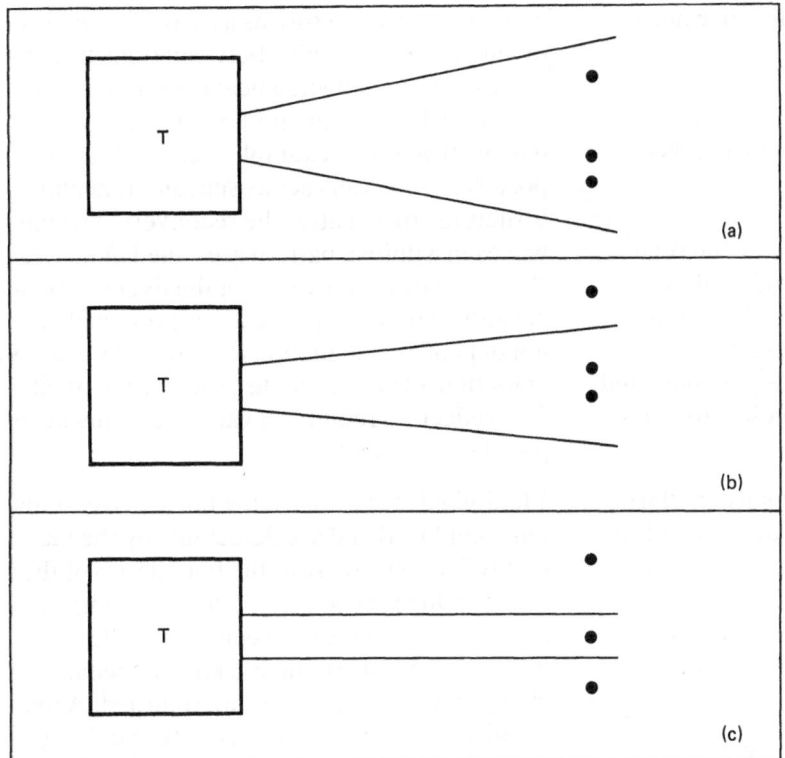

FIGURE 1.5
Lateral resolution. (a) Three point targets displayed as one point. (b) Two point targets shown as one point with better azimuthal resolution due to narrower beam width. (c) Optimal resolution distinguishing two closely spaced targets. [T, transducer]

less than 1 percent of the incident ultrasonic beam energy reflected back to the transducer.

REVERBERATION

The face of the transducer may act as a reflecting surface to returning sound waves. Consequently, the sound beam may bounce back from the surface of the transducer, follow its original course, and, in return, hit the transducer a second time to be displayed on the oscilloscope at a distance twice as far from the transducer as the original echo. This pattern may be repeated with progressively weaker echoes. This phenomenon is called *reverberation* and may produce confusing and troublesome artifacts (Fig. 1.6).

FIGURE 1.6
*Reverberation phenomena.*The face of the transducer acts as a reflecting surface to the returning sound beam. The echo bounced back appears on the oscilloscope as a series of progressively weaker echoes. Note the reverberation artifact in abdominal scanning.

DISTANCE MEASUREMENT OF REFLECTING INTERFACE

By knowing the velocity of sound in the medium being examined and the time it takes for the sonic pulse to strike an interface and return as a reconverted echo, it is possible to measure the distance between the reflecting interface and the transducer. After the sonograph is calibrated for the velocity of sound in the medium

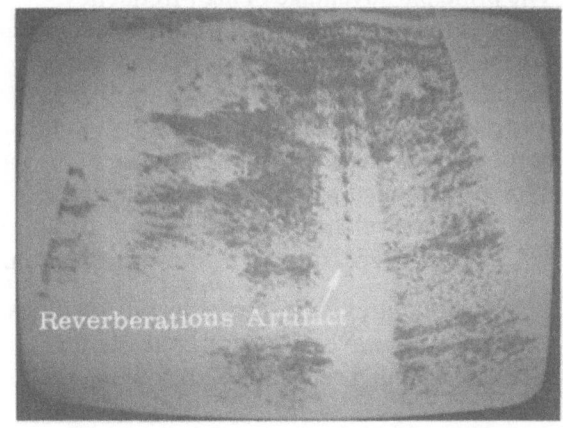

Reverberations Artifact

examined, time is converted to distance automatically.

DIRECTIVITY, REFLECTIVITY, AND TRANSMISSIVITY

Sonography is based on the pulse–echo relationship. Short electric pulses produced by a generator are converted by a transducer into bursts of acoustic energy. The sound beam emitted proceeds in a typical divergent path and produces different echoes, depending upon interacting media.

High-frequency ultrasound has many similarities to light energy. In its course of travel, ultrasound will be reflected and refracted when it strikes an interface between two acoustically different media. If physiologic and geometric conditions are suitable, diffraction also occurs.

Reflection of ultrasound depends on the acoustic impedance mismatch of two media. The greater the difference in impedance, the greater the reflection. That portion of the sound wave not reflected is transmitted through the medium. If the incident beam is not perpendicular to the interface, sound will be reflected and refracted, depending on the angle of incidence (85). The incident beam should be normal to the interface studied to achieve maximum reflection back to the transducer. Snell's law of optical refraction applies to the refraction effect of the incident beam and Huygen's principle of optical diffraction applies to diffraction of the sonic beam.

The principal advantage of high-frequency sound is that it can be aimed toward specific organs. Study by ultrasound is optimal when the beam strikes at an angle perpendicular to the reflecting interface. If the beam is not quite perpendicular to the object of interest, a portion of reflected sound will not return to the crystal. Therefore, correlation between directivity and reflectivity is necessary for a good examination.

Certain structures have high reflecting qualities for ultrasound waves. Flat and concave surfaces are specular reflectors (20), and the re-

converted waves return as a narrow beam. Proper angular relationships between transmitted waves and the reflected beam are required to receive echoes of maximum intensity from this narrow beam. For example, heart valves and posterior cyst walls act as specular reflectors. Structures that scatter the reconverted sound waves in a diffuse pattern are called *diffuse reflectors*. The parenchyma of the liver is a typical diffuse reflector; the echoes produced do not depend on angulation and are usually of low amplitude (45). Adequate examination of diffuse reflectors requires a variety of transducer positions and angles.

Fluid-filled structures in the body cavity transmit sound well and are detectable by the fact that reflection occurs at the boundaries of the cavity, which are areas of differential impedance. The interface between a fluid-filled cavity and bordering tissue is a large impedance change and strong echoes are returned. Acoustic mismatch is much greater between tissue and bone. For example, at the interface between soft tissue and bone, more than 50 percent of the transmitted sound waves will be reflected. At an air–soft tissue interface, 100 percent reflection occurs.

Different organs in the body have different acoustic impedances. Therefore, the transmissivity of sound will change as it travels through various tissues. Every time the transmitted beam of ultrasound strikes an interface, an ultrasonic wave (echo) is reflected back and displayed on an oscilloscope. The greater the acoustic impedance mismatch at the interface between two media, the greater the reflection. Consequently, in heterogeneous media, many echoes are produced; in homogeneous media there are few or no echoes. Therefore, heterogeneous structures are said to be echogenic, whereas homogeneous regions are echo-free or anechoic. A fluid-filled cavity is homogeneous and thus echo free. Fluid-filled cysts and solid masses are differentiated by the absence or presence of echo-producing interfaces within a lesion. This principle is used to diagnose pericardial effusions, ascites, and normal blood pools, such as the aorta.

The acoustic impedance of bone and high atomic number elements is very great, while that of air is low. Therefore, the incident beam at a soft tissue – air interface is totally reflected. Since there is no penetration, lung scanning with ultrasound is impossible at the present time. At soft tissue – bone interfaces, significant quantities of ultrasound are absorbed. Thus, the ribs may produce some difficulty when the liver or spleen is scanned. The bony structures of children, however, cause fewer problems because these structures are smaller and contain less calcium.

DISPLAY MODES

The reflected echoes may be displayed by A-mode, B-mode, B-scan, or M-mode.

A-MODE (AMPLITUDE MODE)

The A-mode ultrasound system displays the electrically converted echo pattern as a vertical deflection (Fig. 1.7a). The amplitude of each deflection is proportional to the reflected energy received by the transducer. The deflections occur at different points on a calibrated tracing, corresponding to the distance of the reflecting surface from the face of the transducer. The number, shape, location, and amplitude of the

FIGURE. 1.7
Display modes. (a) A-mode. Echo producing interfaces produce vertical deflections proportional to echo amplitude. (b) B-scanning. Vertical deflections converted into dots of brightness may be used for scanning. Brightness of dots is proportional to echo amplitude. (c) M-mode. Motion of objects recorded by moving the B-mode tracing along the time axis. [T, transducer]

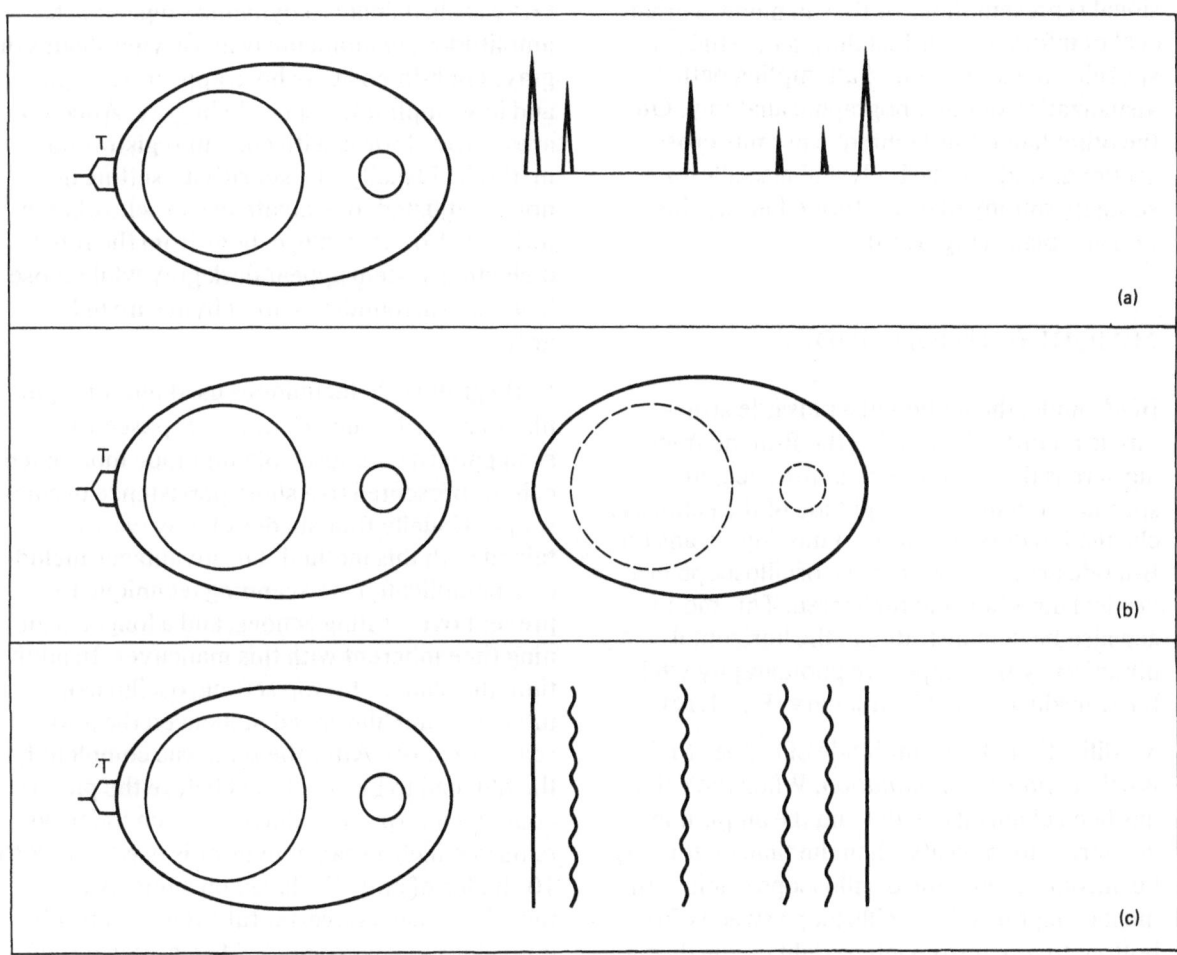

echo spikes furnish detailed information of the structure examined. The horizontal distance between registered echoes is proportional to the depth of the tissue which produced reflection.

B-MODE (BRIGHTNESS MODE)

With B-mode, the echoes are displayed on the oscilloscope as a series of dots and lines, the brightness of which varies with the intensity of the reflected waves, since the echoes are projected as a linear series of bright dots (Fig. 1.7b). The second dimension of the oscilloscope can be used for acoustic section or sonolaparotomy of an organ by moving the transducer in the desired planes. This technique is called *B-scan mode*. Consequently, a single sonolaparotomy produces a two-dimensional representation. In B-scan mode, a great deal of information is lost during the study of a specific area as a result of attempting better visualization of the topographic anatomy. On the other hand, this technique permits cross-sectional study of the body and also allows sonolaparotomy to be performed in any direction and plane (Fig. 1.7b).

M-MODE (MOTION MODE)

In M-mode, the motion of a pulsatile structure is recorded by moving the B-mode tracing across the oscilloscope at preselected speeds. Actually, the amplitude of the echoes is changed to dots. The dots of moving organs on B-mode are swept across the oscilloscope in a vertical direction and registered. This motion can also be demonstrated in the horizontal direction by time exposure photography while the transducer is held stationary (Fig. 1.7c).

Modification of the amplitude of echoes to dots is called *intensity modulation*. When the echo has been changed to a dot and the amplitude converted to intensity, then the time factor may be introduced into the oscilloscope tracing. In most echograms the oscilloscope sweeps from bottom to top or from left to right on the display tube. When the M-mode sweeping has a vertical and horizontal motion, one dimension can be used for time and the other for distance. The tracing can be displayed on a regular TV monitor as a black and white or a gray scale by using a scan converter.

The M-mode presentation may be recorded on polaroid film or on a cathode ray tube. A strip chart recorder affords better detail.

GRAY-SCALE IMAGING

Conventional B-scan systems use threshold detection to register echoes on a phosphor storage oscilloscope screen. Echoes above a certain amplitude are displayed as dots of constant intensity, while echoes of lesser amplitude are not displayed.

Gray scale displays a dynamic range of echo amplitudes simultaneously as varying shades of gray. High-intensity echoes appear dark gray and low amplitude echoes light gray. Anechoic areas are colorless with current registration methods. Usually, the sensitivity setting need not be adjusted to evaluate tissue echo characteristics. For example, echoes from the renal collecting system appear dark gray while those from the surrounding parenchyma are light gray.

Early gray-scale techniques used photographic film to record scans. Film was exposed to a scan pattern composed of amplitude modulated echoes presented to a short-persistence oscilloscope. Usually four shades of gray were obtained with this method. Disadvantages included a complicated arc scanning technique to prevent overwriting echoes, and a longer scanning time inherent with this maneuver. In addition, the camera F-stop setting, oscilloscope intensity, and film speed influenced the gray-scale effect (8). After the scan was completed, the film had to be developed before the picture could be interpreted. Current commercial systems in which a scan converter is used offer 8 to 10 shades of gray displayed on a television tube. The scan converter tube detects all echo intensities and is connected to a closed circuit

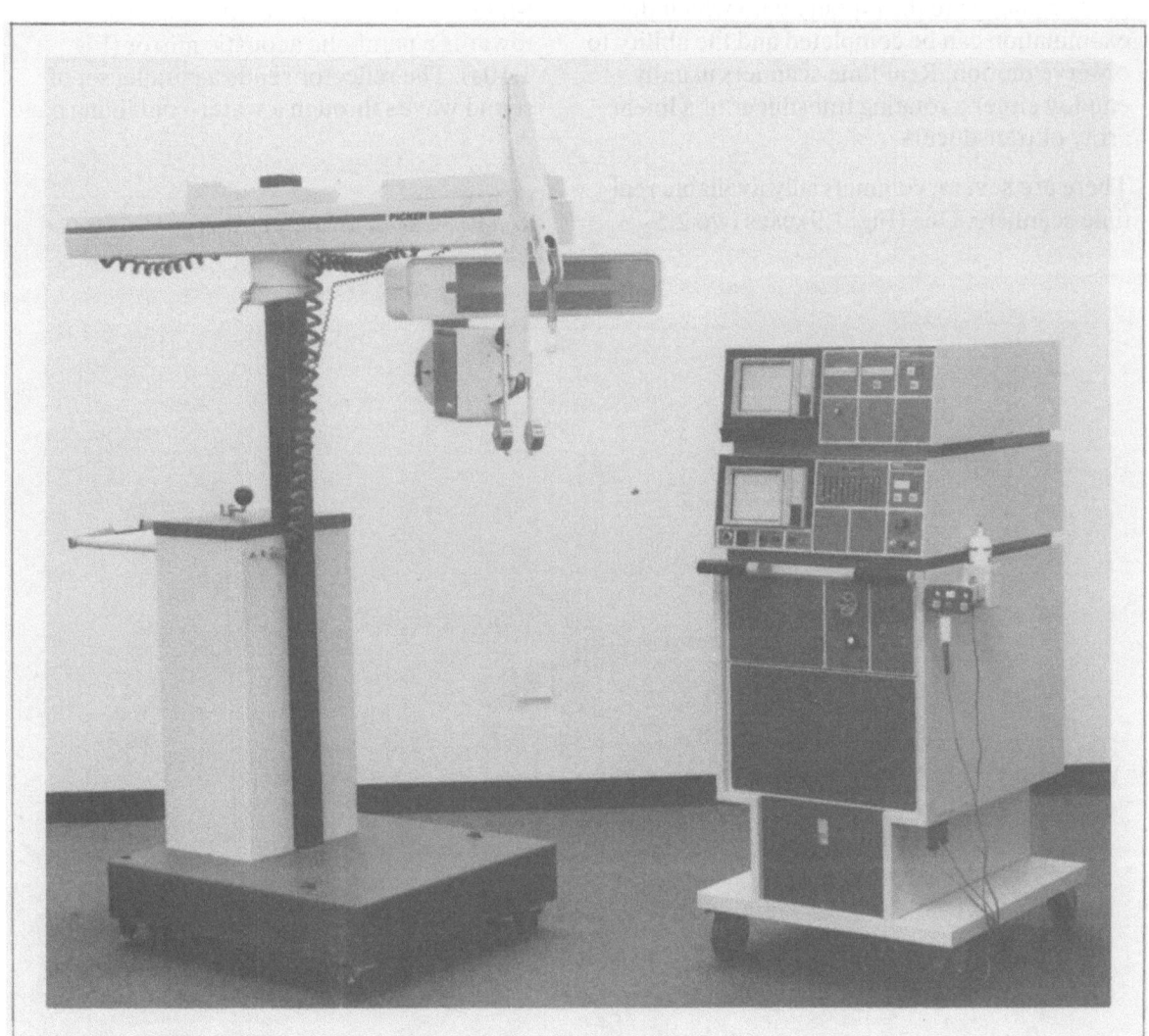

FIGURE 1.8
Contact diagnostic ultrasound scanner (courtesy of Picker Corporation).

television system providing an instant visual display of the area scanned. The technique is the same as for conventional B-scanning methods. Scanning time is reduced due to better resolution and simultaneous display of weak and strong echoes, eliminating the need to vary sensitivity settings during sectioning. The image developed on the monitor tube may then be recorded with polaroid 70 or 35 mm film. Moderate differentiation of signal processing enhances contrast at tissue interfaces (8). Most scan converter systems offer information-processing techniques for postscan image optimization (Fig. 1.8).

REAL-TIME SCANNING

The real-time scanner has added new dimensions to the scope of information available from ultrasonic examination. This modality has been applied to numerous areas of the body (56,84,86). The two main advantages of real-time scanning are the rapidity with which the examination can be completed and the ability to observe motion. Real-time scanners usually employ either a rotating transducer or a linear array of transducers.

There are several commercially available real-time scanners. One (Fig. 1.9) uses two 2.5- MHz transducers that emit ultrasonic beams towards a parabolic acoustic mirror (Fig. 1.10a). The reflector sends a parallel set of sound waves through a water-containing bag

FIGURE 1.9
Real-time scanner (courtesy of Siemens Company).

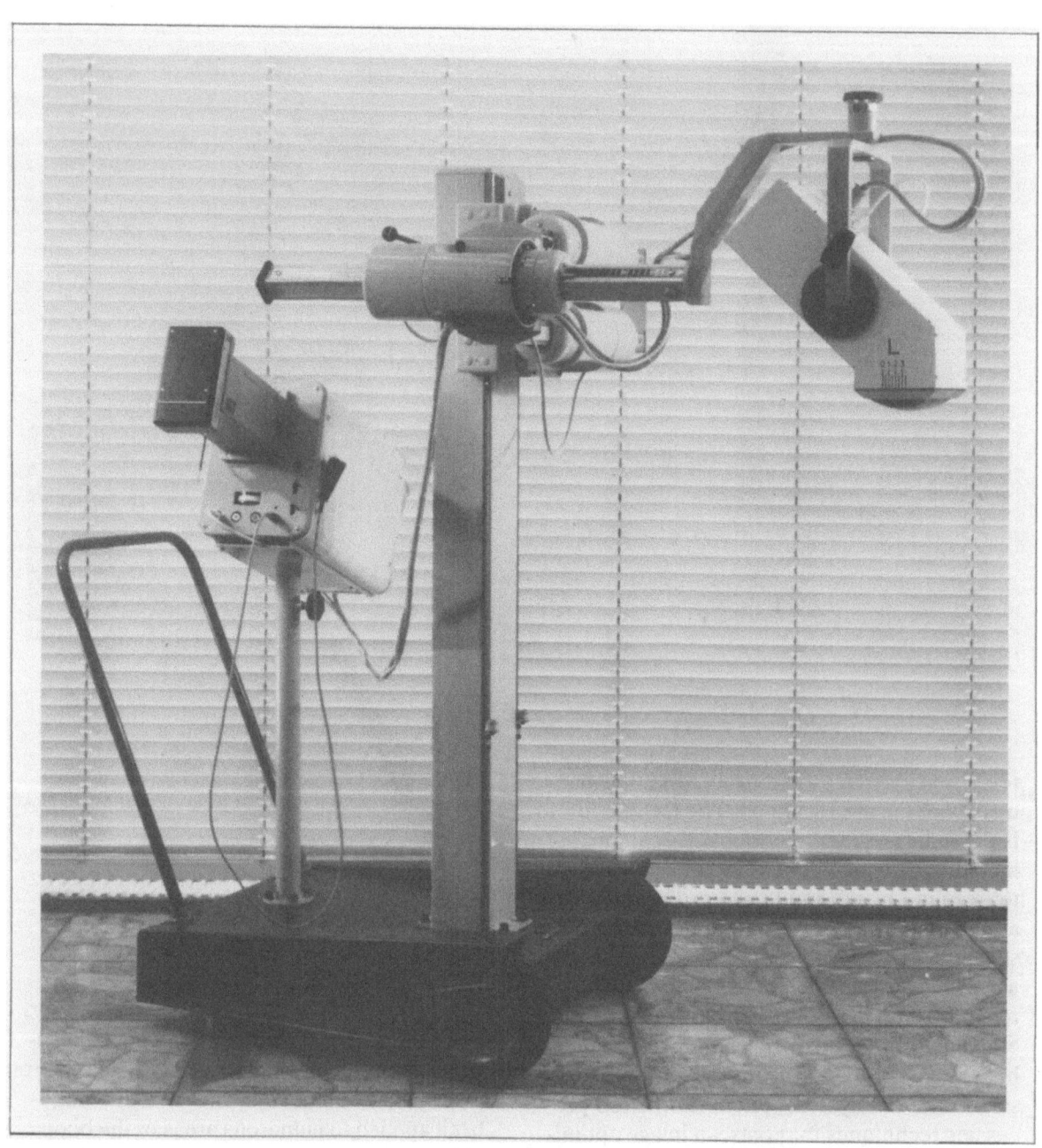

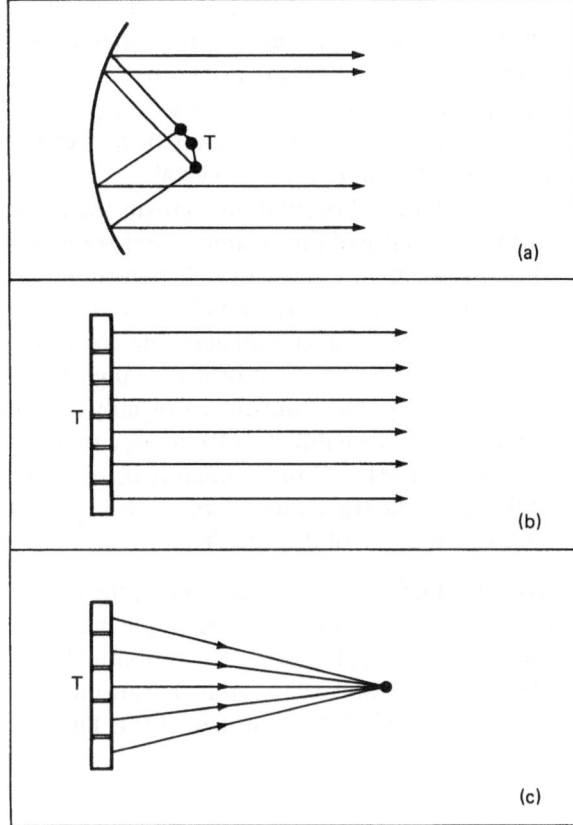

FIGURE 1.10
Real-time scanning systems. (a) Rotating transducer reflects sound waves from parabolic surface to generate parallel beam. (b) Linear Transducer Array. Multiple transducers being pulsed in sequence to produce parallel beam. (c) Phased Linear Array. Variable wavefront generated by coordinated pulsing of each transducer element. [T, transducer]

applied to the body surface. A gel is used as a coupling agent. The scanning field is covered 15 times per second and the sectional view studied is about 14 cm in length and 20 cm in depth. This field is built up to approximately 120 lines within 70 msec. The width of the section is a few millimeters.

The unit produces instantaneous sectional images and displays them simultaneously on an oscilloscope and television monitor. This immediate and continuous presentation makes it possible to visually record movement of a desired structure. Without shifting the applicator head, parallel sectional scans can be taken up to 3.5 cm laterally by remote control of the motion

of the transducer mounted within the applicator head.

The linear array scanner, in which the applicator has a linear array of 64 transducers, firing four at a time, to produce approximately 60 lines of information (Fig. 1.10b), has recently been developed.

Both machines are equipped with depth compensation controls which amplify the near, far, or overall field. Another device adjusts the shades of gray on the monitor.

Linear transducer arrays may be electronically phased by pulsing each of the multiple transducer crystals as a separate unit. The wave front formed follows the pattern of transducer excitation. The wave pattern may be made to produce a sector scan with a variable scan angle up to 90°. The wave front may also be focused to different depths. Resolution with current systems varies (Fig. 1.10c).

EQUIPMENT AND PRACTICAL ASPECTS

CONSTRUCTION OF AN
ULTRASOUND INSTRUMENT

The essential part of a sonographic unit consists of the following elements:

1. *Transducer.* The transducer acts as a sender and receiver of sonic waves. It functions as a receiver 99.9 percent of the time.
2. *Transmitter.* The transmitter regulates the sonic waves through the transducer. A timer in the transmitter controls the frequency and duration of ultrasonic pulses emitted by the transducer.
3. *Receiver.* Returning echoes reconverted through the transducer to electrical impulses are picked up by the receiver and signal amplifier.
4. *Signal amplifier.* The signal amplifier, located between the receiver and cathode ray tube, increases the voltage of the signal.
5. *Cathode ray tube.* The cathode ray tube receives the amplified impulses of

the returning echo. The processed impulses are displayed on the cathode ray tube or oscilloscope.

TRANSDUCERS

COMPONENTS

The transducer has a lead zirconate crystal with piezoelectric properties and can expand and contract in response to electric pulses. (Fig. 1.1a and b). The piezoelectric crystal has a small cylindrical shape and is generally 1 to 2 cm wide and 1 mm thick. The electrodes providing the electric potential are connected to both sides of the crystal. The vibrating crystal

causes compressions and rarefactions in all directions. To provide an undirectional ultrasonic beam, a backing material is used to absorb the waves in unwanted directions. The backing material acts as an acoustic as well as a mechanical damper for the crystal.

The frequency of oscillation controls the resolution capability of the system. After transmission, the acoustic energy of reflected sound is reconverted into electric impulses for data analysis, since the same crystal generates electric currents when exposed to returning high-frequency waves. The transducers usually used in clinical work have different frequency ranges, from 1 to 15 MHz. Approximately 0.1 percent of the time, the transducer acts as a transmitter and 99.9 percent of the time it acts as a receiver.

To vary the frequency of the sound, the transducer must be changed. For example, a frequency of 2.25 MHz is used in abdominal studies. For echocardiography, a transducer frequency of 3.5 MHz is utilized (24). The

FIGURE 1.11
Transducer beam patterns. (a) Nonfocused transducer. Parallel wavefront forms the near field. Divergent beam in far field. (b) Focused transducer. Narrowest beam width at focal zone. (c) Collimated transducer. Elongated near field and less far field beam divergence. [T, transducer]

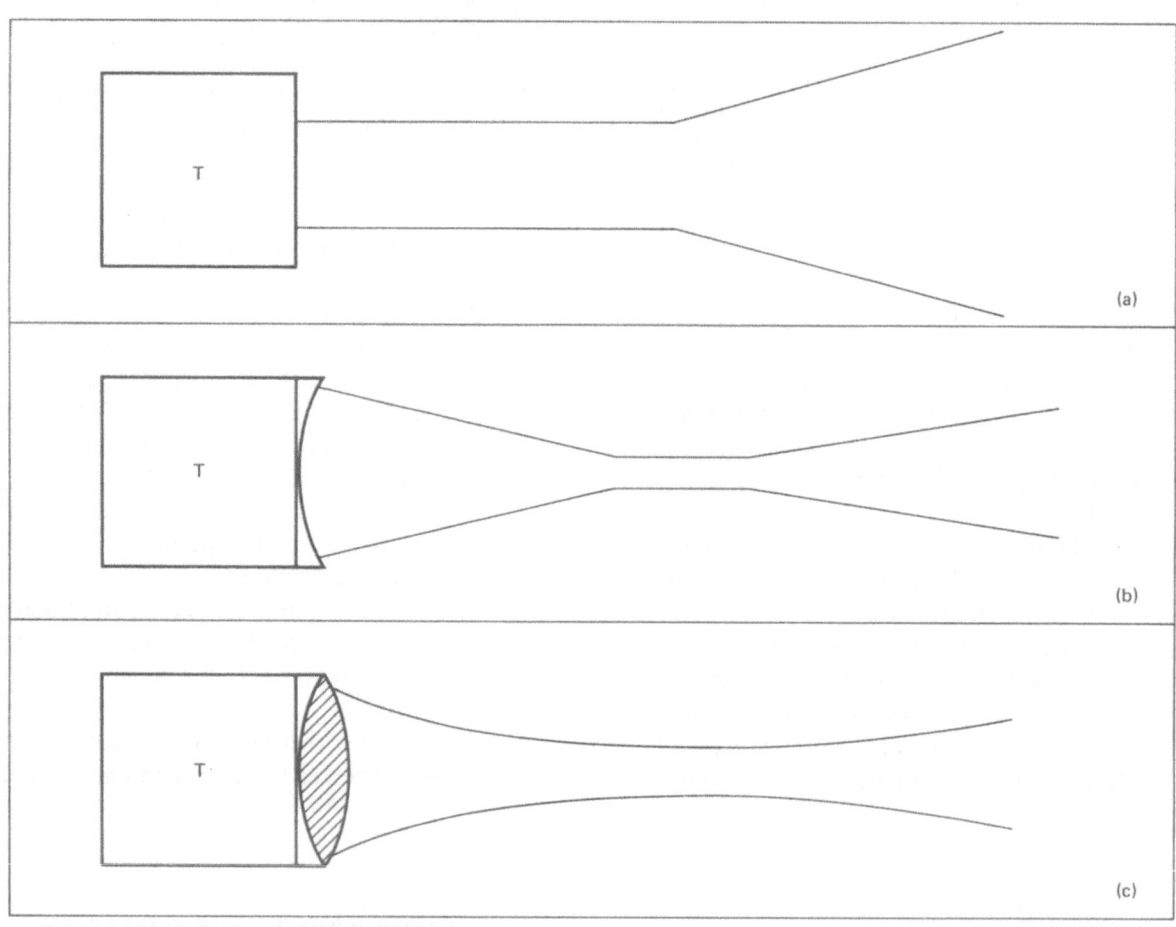

characteristics of the system depend on the frequency of the transducer and the choice of frequency depends on the region to be studied(24). Transducers of low frequency have longer wavelengths, resulting in greater beam penetration and better depth of study. However, increasing the wavelength decreases the resolution of the system. High frequency offers high resolution. In ophthalmology, the transducer frequency varies from 7.5 to 15 MHz. As a result, the higher frequency provides optimal definition of small objects but the depth of penetration is limited.

MOUNTING

The disc of piezoelectric crystal in the transducer has a suitable mounting arrangement for optimal resolution. (2,3,15). To produce continuous waves a thin layer of a matching wave is used to improve the sensitivity (24). In the back of the transducer is a loading or backing material, which absorbs sound energy directed or transmitted backward. Consequently, the quality and shape of forward energy, especially those of short pulses, are improved.

NEAR FIELD AND FAR FIELD

Divergence of the beam from the transducer is of extreme importance. In a circular transducer, the beam emitted from the face is cylindrical. During the course of propagation, the sound waves run parallel for a certain distance and then gradually begin to diverge. That portion of the beam close to and parallel with the transducer is called the *near field* and that from the divergent point is called the *far field* (Fig. 1.11a, b, and c). At the end of the near field, the intensity of sound is maximal in the axis of the beam. Thus, maximum information is obtained when the object is located in the near field because the sound beam is parallel to the transducer and more perpendicular to the target. Consequently, the intensity of the reconverted echo is greater.

OPTIMAL CRYSTAL SIZE

To increase the resolution of the ultrasonic beam (20), its width should be as small as possible. To enlarge the near field and obtain better information, the size of the crystal is increased or wavelength decreased. Reducing the diameter of the crystal narrows the width of the beam but decreases the length of the near field and increases the divergent angle of the far field (20).

To obtain the optimum size of the transducer crystal, the beam width should be constructed in such a way that the near field is half the desired operating range of the transducer. To obtain higher resolution, frequency should be increased. In practice, the highest frequency consistent with maximum penetration for the required study is utilized (Fig. 1.12a, b and c).

FOCUSED

Resolution can also be improved by using a focused or collimated transducer to reduced beam width within the focal zone. By applying a focusing lens with a concave surface, the focus of the ultrasonic beam will be narrowed to a predetermined distance from the face of the transducer (Fig. 1.11b and c). The focused transducer has helped to improve resolution of deep abdominal structures.

FUNCTION

As previously described, piezoelectric crystals emit ultrasound pulses as short as 1 μsec. After the sonic burst has been emitted, the transducer then acts as a receiver, picking up the reflected sonic waves. After this period of time, another burst of ultrasound is emitted and the cycle repeated. There are different types of transducers, some of which are described below.

TRANSDUCER	USE
2.25 MHz	General purpose
13 mm diameter, focused	scanning
3.5 MHz	Pediatrics
13 mm diameter, focused	
2.25 MHz	
13 mm diameter, nonfocused	
3.17 mm hole	Biopsy A-mode
2.25 MHz	
13 mm diameter, nonfocused	
3.17 mm hole	Biopsy B-scan
2.25 MHz	Deep-tissue scanning
19 mm diameter, long internal focus	

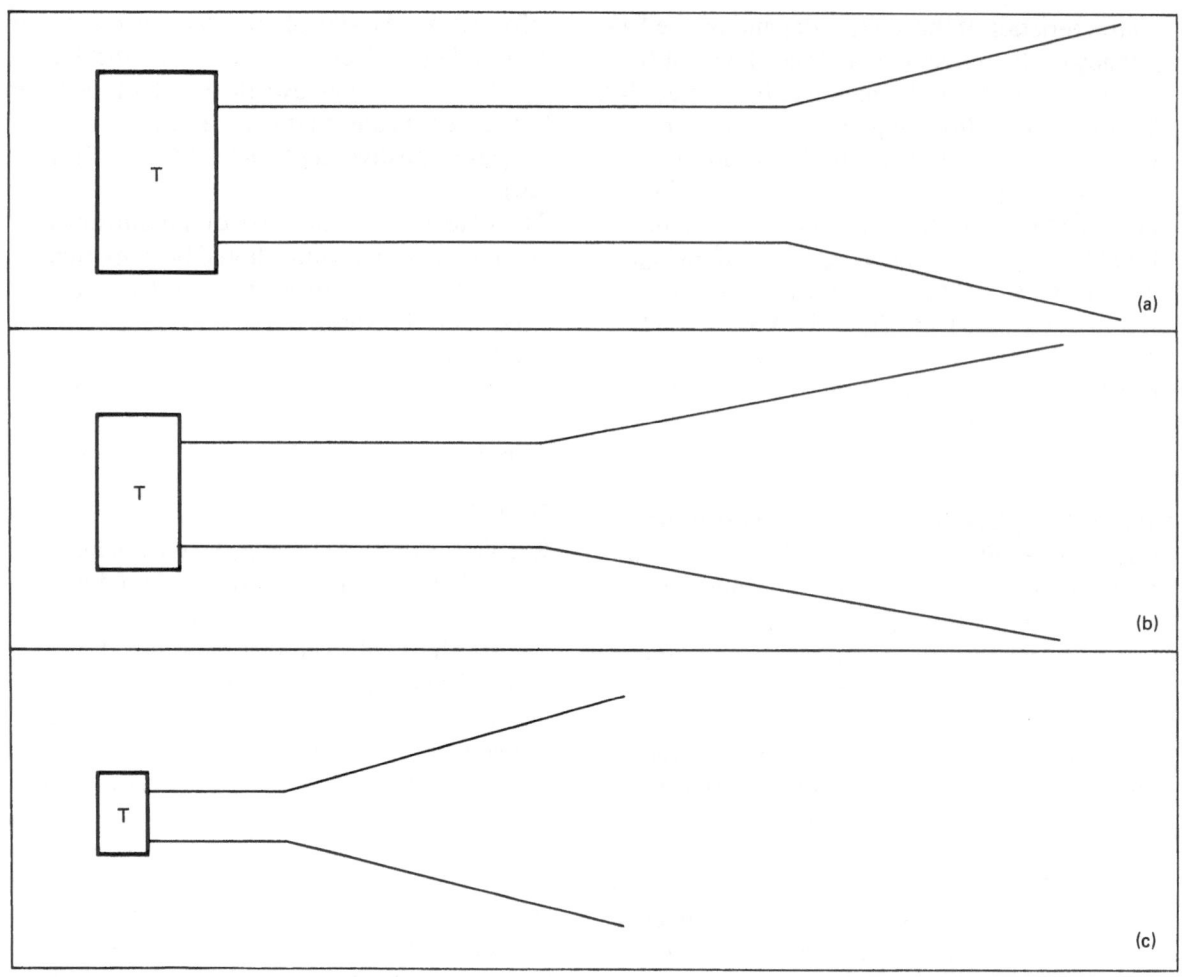

FIGURE 1.12
Beam width and crystal size. (a) Wide crystal with long near field. (b) Medium crystal with shorter near field (c) Narrow crystal with short near field and great beam divergence in the far field. [T, transducer]

PULSE CHARACTERISTICS AND DAMPING SYSTEM

The optimal spatial pulse length is between 1 and 2½ cycles. The excited crystal has a tendency to oscillate for a long time, producing a prolonged spatial pulse length too long to provide adequate axial resolution. The damping system controls crystal oscillation by mechanical and electronic means (Fig. 1.13a, b, and c). Damping may be adjusted manually or built into the electronic circuitry. Overdamping produces a short spatial pulse length and the pulse may lack sufficient energy to be useful. Thus, a properly spaced pulse depends on a well-adjusted damping system.

SIGNAL PROCESSING

Reconverted ultrasonic echoes produce an electric impulse when they reach the transducer crystal. This impulse is transmitted as an amplified RF (15,24) (Radio Frequency) signal into the system. The RF mode appears as a series of signals above and below the baseline of the oscilloscope (Fig. 1.14a and b). Amplification increases the size of the signal without changing the information and is manually adjustable (gain control). Further modification depends on specific clinical use. Generally, after amplification, the waveform is rectified to remove all negative

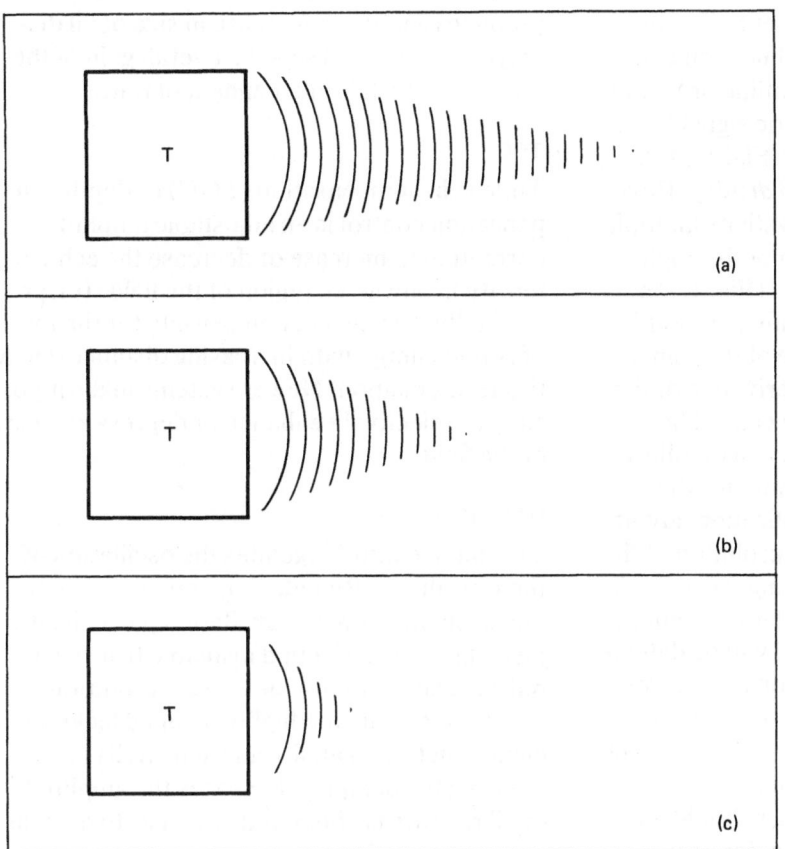

FIGURE 1.13
Damping effect. (a) Underdamping resulting in multiple oscillations of transducer crystal. (b) Proper damping producing optimal spatial pulse length. (c) Overdamping with insufficient pulse cycles. [T, transducer]

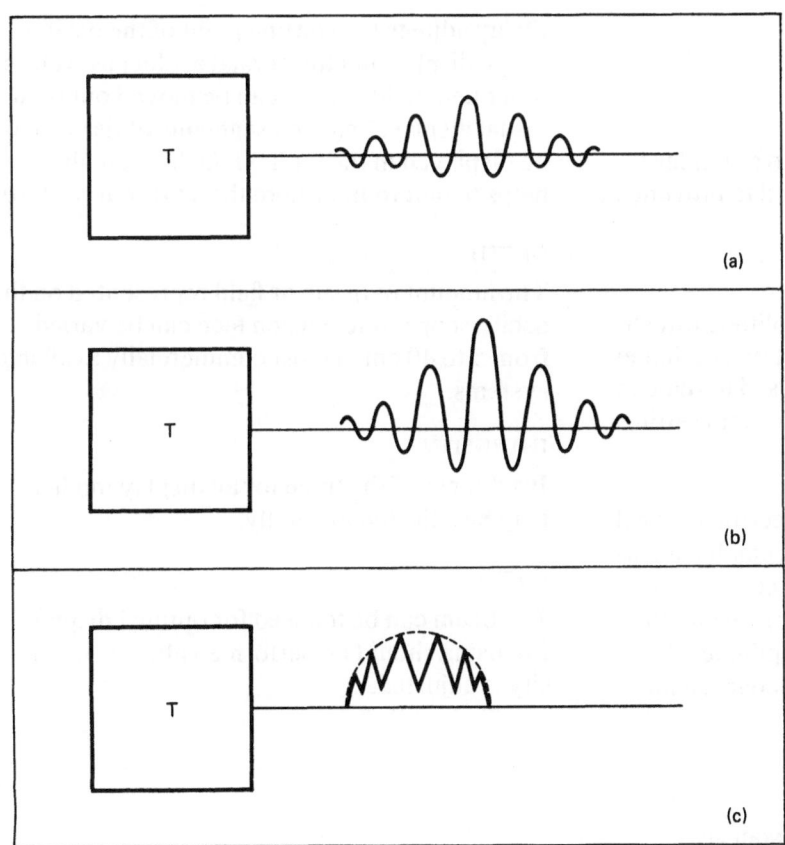

FIGURE 1.14
Signal processing. (a) RF signal produced by incoming echo on transducer crystal. (b) Amplification of RF signal. (c) Rectification of RF signal and envelope detection. [T, transducer]

components so that only the upper half of the signal is presented. Further modification can be accomplished so that only the outline or boundary of the upper half of the electric signal is presented as an *envelope detection* (Fig. 1.14c). This presentation is called *video display*. Envelope detection or video display with its multiple peaks can be converted into a smooth, single, large peak called the *video signal* (Fig. 1.15a). This signal may be further amplified or modified by accentuating the leading edge of the signal (Fig. 1.15b) by taking the first derivative of the video signal that produces a thin echo. The small negative phase (Fig. 1.15b and c) following the initial signal further accentuates the leading edge of the echo by rectification, giving finer echoes and enhancing the resolution of the system. Another step in processing the video is to add a reject level so that only large amplitude echoes above a certain threshold will be detected (Fig 1.16 a, b, and c). Rejection is very important to eliminate unnecessary echoes and electric noise or "grass" (Fig. 1.16b). However, certain low-level echoes are required for optimal information. The sonographer should adjust the rejection level, as needed, for proper ultrasonic examination.

MAIN SYSTEM CONTROL

POWER SWITCH

An off–on switch is connected to a standard 110 V outlet. The line is grounded to prevent an electric hazard.

REJECT

The reject control varies the amplitude threshold required to record an echo. It discriminates against low-level echoes and is used to remove "grass"-like interference at higher gain settings.

GAIN

The gain control amplifies the electronic signal of the received echo. Some units employ an attenuation system to achieve this effect. Two types of gain are available — near gain and total gain. Near gain increases the amplitude of echoes in the near field. Total or coarse gain

produces a uniform increase in size of all displayed signals, and sets the overall gain of the receiver, which is independent of range.

TGC

Time gain compensation (TGC) or depth compensation control is an adjustable amplitude correction to increase or decrease the echo intensity in any given region of the field. It was originally designed to compensate for the loss of sound energy with increasing distance due to tissue attenuation. Newer systems make it possible to selectively enhance or depress any part of the field.

DAMPING

The damp control regulates the oscillation of the transducer. By reducing or damping transducer ringing from the excitation pulse, it adjusts the cycles of sound available from each pulse. A shorter pulse increases resolution; however, a beam too highly damped lacks sufficient penetrating ability and sensitivity. Increasing the damping decreases the amplitude of all recorded echoes and is similar to decreasing the total gain.

DELAY

Delay adjusts the starting point of the oscilloscope display and the crystal artifact as well as other near field echoes can be moved out of the visual display. Selected segments of tissue may be displayed in the far field. Delay actually helps to determine where the TGC curve starts.

DEPTH

The amount of tissue or field represented on the oscilloscope or television face can be varied from 5 to 40 cm in most commercially available systems.

INTENSITY

Brightness of the trace for all display modes may be adjusted manually.

FOCUS

The beam can be focused for optimal display. Focusing should be performed after its intensity is adjusted.

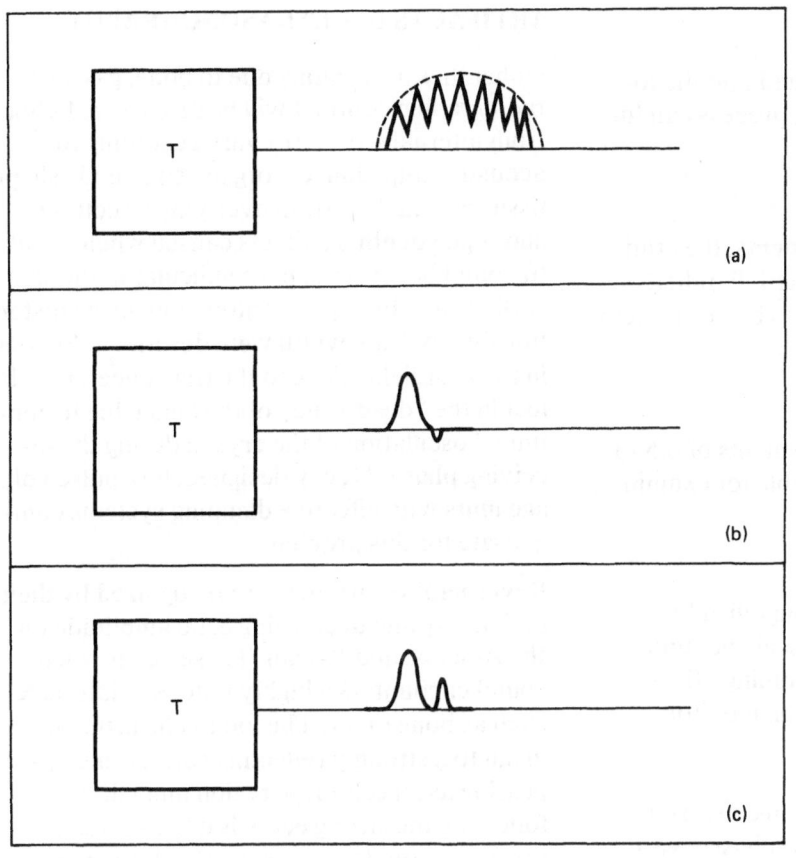

FIGURE 1.15
Signal processing. (a) Envelope detection of rectified RF signal. (b) Leading edge display or differentiation of signal. (c) Rectification and amplification of signal for oscilloscope display. [T, transducer]

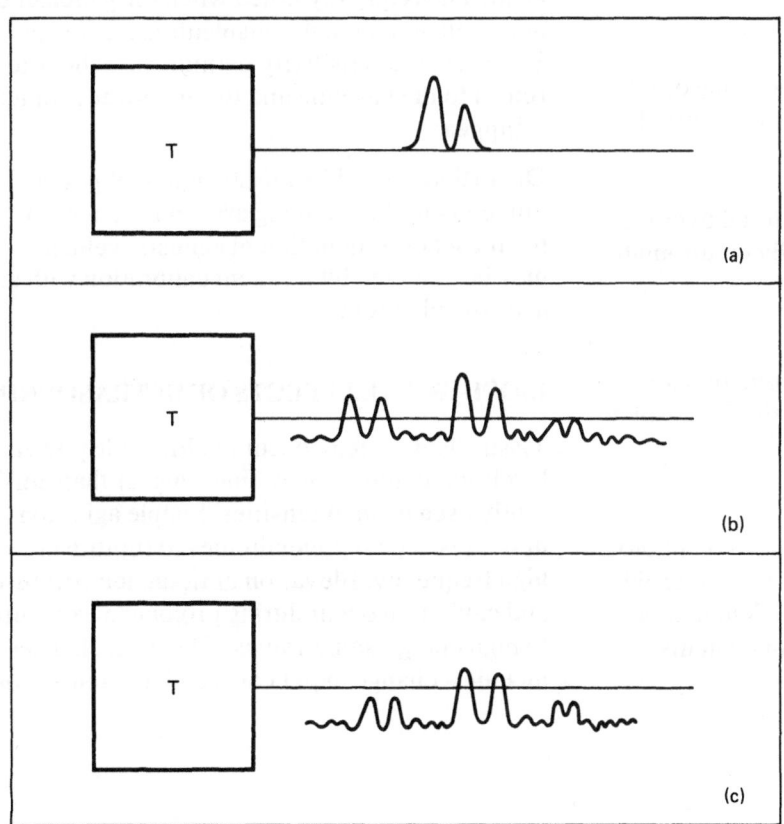

FIGURE 1.16
Rejection. (a) RF signal. (b) Amplified signal with unwanted echoes and electrical noise. (c) Elevation of baseline echo threshold displaying only amplified signal. [T, transducer]

19

ASTIGMATISM

Astigmatism may be incorporated into the focus system so that the focusing process can further be refined.

GRATICULE

A reference scale for measurements, the graticule can be adjustably illuminated. Parallel, transverse, and longitudinal lines form a pattern of squares.

SCALE

The field may be varied in increments of 0.5 to 3 cm per square, which is valuable for examining smaller organs.

MAGNIFICATION

The echoes displayed can be magnified by either rescanning on a smaller scale per unit square or by electronically "zooming" the image presented on the television monitor.

CONTRAST ENHANCEMENT

Newer gray-scale units offer scan converter tubes that make it possible to emphasize various shades of gray to maximize the information display.

ERASE

An erase switch clears the oscilloscope or television tube so that a new scan can be started.

CENTER

The scanning beam must be centered over the oscilloscope field, either manually or automatically.

DIGITAL READ OUT

A computer "types" patient information and scan identification directly onto the TV display, which may then be photographed.

RECORDING

A permanent record can be obtained on photographic film of the 35 mm, 70 mm, or polaroid type. X-ray film can also be used. Video tape systems may be adapted for permanent displays.

ARTIFACTS IN ULTRASONOGRAPHY

Difficulties in scanning due to bone, gas, and radiographic contrast will be discussed. Echoes from internal structures vary according to acoustic impedance, organ size and shape, tissue attenuation from overlying structures, and organ depth. Artifacts caused when the ultrasound beam is not perpendicular to the skin surface, and by organ contour and image distortion due to beam width were described. Echoes in the near field, close to the transducer, may be lost in the "dead zone" of the beam due to continued oscillation of the crystal during the receiving phase. Newly designed, low-pulse voltage units with effective damping systems compensate for this problem.

Reverberation artifacts are recognized by their periodicity and decreasing echo amplitude on the A-scope and B-scan. These occur when sound encounters a highly reflecting interface, such as bone or air. The loud-echo artifact, distal to a strongly reflecting surface and appearing as an echo-free region immediately following the strong echo, is due to crystal reverberation. It is noted on the A-scope as echoes elevated from the baseline (4). This artifact is frequently noted when the gallbladder and edematous renal transplants are scanned. Lowering the sensitivity permits the echoes to return to the baseline and the echo-free artifact disappears.

Distortion caused by misalignment of potentiometers in the scanning arm and changes in the preset determination of acoustic velocity may be detected by frequent calibration with an acoustic phantom.

BIOPHYSICAL EFFECTS OF ULTRASOUND

Tissue damage may occur at ultrasonic power levels many thousand of times higher than currently used beam intensities. Simple agitation may cause cellular membranes to rupture at high frequency. Elevation of tissue temperature and cavitation occur during prolonged exposure to high energy sonic waves. Chemical changes include a change in pH caused by the release of radicles and increased tissue oxidation rates. Also noted are increased membrane permeability and greater enzymatic activity. Since ultrasound is nonionizing, cumulative effects are not to be expected (55).

GENETIC EFFECTS OF ULTRASOUND

The increased use of ultrasound in fetal and maternal disorders and its recent application to the male testis requires investigation into the potential genetic hazards of clinical sonography. An excellent *in vivo* study of mice gonads insonated at levels up to 20 times the intensity of currently used ultrasound energy intensities revealed no evidence that dominant lethal mutations or sterility is induced in male mice. Follow-up for eight weeks demonstrated no drop in testis weight or sperm count and no induction of translocations or chromosome fragments in spermatocytes (55). Although the risk of genetic derangements from ultrasound appears to be slight, its carcinogenic effect may not have been fully evaluated in humans at this early stage in the widespread application of ultrasonography to the general population.

PRACTICAL ASPECTS OF SONOLAPAROTOMY

In sonolaparotomy proper direction of the beam towards a specific organ is essential. Familiarity with ultrasonic sectional anatomy and knowledge of anatomic pathology and surface topography are extremely important. Comprehension of organ relationships and their normal ultrasonic pattern is necessary to evaluate the extent of disease and the involvement of adjacent structures by pathologic processes.

PATIENT PREPARATION

In most instances there is no need for patient preparation. In obstetric and gynecologic examinations the bladder should be distended to delineate pelvic organs and to increase the penetration of the ultrasonic beam. To study the pancreas, it is preferable that the patient be NPO since it may be necessary to insert a nasogastric tube to suction out gastric air or instill gasless water to distend the stomach and outline the duodenal contour.

Scanning causes no discomfort for the patient and in many situations is similar to fluoroscopy in that the patient must be positioned properly and the image on the screen monitored constantly. After the area to be scanned is exposed, mineral oil is usually applied to the skin surface to prevent an air gap, which would markedly reflect sound between the transducer and abdominal wall. Complete contact between the rubber diaphragm of the real-time scanner and the skin surface is obtained by using an ultrasonic gel.

DUTIES OF THE TECHNOLOGIST

The sonographer should clearly understand the various methods of examination and proper control settings of the scanning machine used.

Patience and search are basic to good ultrasonography. The method of study changes the quality of echo display. Each type of commercially available instrument has its characteristic image production. For this reason, each unit functions with its own criteria, and the art of sonography is to extract maximum information from a specific unit.

However, certain techniques and criteria are essential for basic studies. These include the sonographer's familiarity with the following technical considerations:

1. Arrangement of a proper TGC curve on the oscilloscope for the study of a specific organ.
2. Selection of the proper transducer.
3. Familiarity with a system of identification.
4. Changing the gain setting as needed.
5. Selection of the rate of sectoring.
6. Knowledge of the types of scanning (linear, compound, arc, or sector).

7. Study of the patient in multiple positions.
8. Maintenance of a minimum of eight shades of gray in gray-scale units.
9. Familiarity with the use of real-time scanning.
10. Knowledge of the ultrasonic limitations of sonography.
11. Detection of through transmission pattern in combined A-mode and B-mode for better evaluation of pathology (31).

PHYSICIAN PARTICIPATION

Sonography is similar to creating a painting. The art of the operator is to display the echoes from a lesion and demonstrate its shape, location, and texture. Sonography is far more delicate than fluoroscopy in that pathology detection and physician performance are more demanding. The examiner must make a final interpretation before the procedure is terminated. A specifically trained nurse-technician can perform the study; however the physician-in-charge should be in constant attendance for consultation and to interpret specific findings shown on the polaroid. For example, during a routine study of the liver for metastases from an unknown source, a hypernephroma of the upper pole of the right kidney may be incidentally discovered.

POSITIONING THE TRANSDUCER

The transducer acts as a transmitter and receiver and the time between sonic emission and returned echo is a measure of the depth of the reflecting surface. Maximum reflection is achieved when the organ of interest lies perpendicular to the sonic beam. Any degree of tilt of the transducer or reflector diminishes the intensity of the echo, and the signal may even be lost.

In certain cases, difficulty in positioning the transducer and factors such as obesity can attenuate the returned ultrasound.

The art of ultrasonography is to be aware of target displacement from the transducer and make corrections. Selection of a proper scanning speed is important if every echo produced is to be recorded (34). If the speed of scanning is too fast, many reflected echoes will be missed by the receiving transducer. If the speed is too slow, artifactual echoes may be produced because the reflected sound will have a higher signal concentration in specific areas at a given period of time. The rate of transducer motion should be constant regardless of the scanning speed. When a normal technique is not applicable, other variations must be devised. Changes may be made in the transducer, patient position, scanning plane, or scanning mode. For example, 1-MHz transducer may salvage a study in which a 2.25-MHz transducer cannot penetrate excess subcutaneous fat, in renal

FIGURE 1.17
Types of scanning. (a) Linear Scan. Sound beam at right angles to the skin surface. (b) Sector Scan. Transducer rotated about a fixed axis. (c) Compound Scan. Combination of linear and sector scan. [T, transducer]

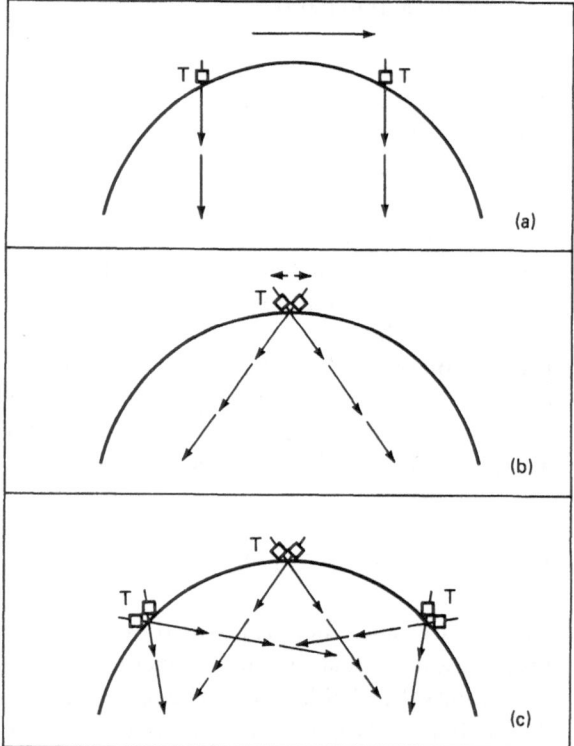

scanning hyperextension of the patient may permit better delineation of the kidney, multiple scanning planes are generally necessary to visualize the entire pancreas, and minimal ascites may not be detected on routine supine B-scanning but application of the A-mode transducer to the dependent anterior abdominal wall will demonstrate as little as 100 ml of free fluid. M-mode and real-time scanners may be used to verify the pulsation of a vascular structure.

TYPES OF SCANNING

There are several types of scanning:

- A. Manual B-scanning
  1. Linear scan (Fig. 1.17a)
  2. Sector scan (Fig. 1.17b)
  3. Compound scan (Fig. 1.17c)
  4. Arc scan
- B. Automated B-scanning (Octoson)
- C. Real-time scanning

ULTRASONIC IDENTIFICATION

PRINCIPLE OF SECTIONAL SCANNING

Evaluation of ultrasonic studies requires a complete three-dimensional representation of organs and areas of pathologic significance. As the application of ultrasound in medicine increases, more information can be obtained. A precise and accurate identification system makes it easier to interpret an echogram. For this reason special scanning planes are needed to perform the study and to obtain a corresponding sonic pattern to compare with routine radiographs. The system of identification in some ultrasound departments uses the umbilicus as a reference point. In supine positions sectional scanning (transverse and longitudinal) planes are obtained by considering the umbilicus as the zero point. Sections above and to the right of the umbilicus are designated *plus cuts* and sections below and to the left are called *minus sections*. We have been using

a different identification system for upper abdominal sonography to avoid disadvantages of the above system.

Disadvantages of the above identification system are:

1. Correlating sonograms with radiographs. It is necessary, in many instances (especially studies of the upper abdomen), to compare ultrasonic photographs with corresponding radiographs. When the umbilicus is used as a topographic reference point information is not obtained, which can be used to compare studies with ultrasonic sectoral scanning, unless a lead marker is attached to the umbilicus before the patient is exposed to x-ray. The position of the umbilicus varies in many pathologic conditions and even among normal young and old individuals. Indeed, it may be surgically absent. Since it is not a fixed reference point, the exact echogram cannot be reproduced in repeat examination in many pathologic conditions (ascites, abdominal mass, and so forth) after a lapse of time.
2. Absence of a system using prone, decubitus, angled, and oblique scanning planes.

REFERENCE POINTS

Experience has shown that many obstacles present in previous studies would be avoided if a fixed structure in the body was used as a reference point. (32). We use the xiphoid process of the sternum, symphysis pubis, and crest of the ilium as reference points.

AREAS TO BE IDENTIFIED

1. Right upper quadrant. Use the iliac crest as a reference point.
   (a) Right lobe of liver and gallbladder
   (b) Right kidney

(c) Pyloric portion of fluid-filled stomach
(d) First and second portions of fluid-filled duodenum
(e) Part of fluid-filled ascending and transverse colon (Fig. 1.18)
(f) Head of pancreas
(g) Vascular structures with real-time scanner or gray scale
2. Left upper quadrant. Use the iliac crest as a reference point.
(a) Left lobe of liver
(b) Spleen
(c) Left kidney
(d) Fundus and body of fluid-filled stomach
(e) Body of pancreas
(f) Vascular structures with real-time scanner or gray scale
3. Right lower quadrant
(a) Fluid-filled cecum and ascending colon (Fig. 1.19)
(b) Right psoas muscle
4. Left lower quadrant
(a) Fluid-filled part of descending and sigmoid colon
(b) Left psoas muscle

ANTERIOR PROJECTION

ATC — SERIES

In the anterior projections, if a line is drawn between the two iliac crests, it will pass approximately through the plane of the umbilicus. This transcrestal line or plane represents the zero point and is called the *ATC* (Anterior Transcrestal Plane). All sections above are ATC plus (ATC+1, +2, +3) and all sections below this plane are ATC minus (ATC−1, −2, −3). Each number corresponds to the centimeter distance from the ATC plane. In scanning the pancreas, the hilum of the right kidney is localized and oblique sections are made between the hilum of the right kidney and the spleen. These slices are called *KP* (kidney — pancreas) sections. Other vascular landmarks that can be used to localize the pancreas will be discussed in detail in Chapter 4.

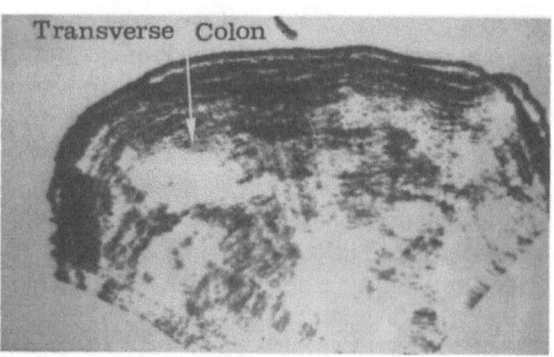

FIGURE 1.18
Supine transverse scan. Transverse echo-free structure below the liver surface. A water enema will show an increase in the size of this zone and distinguish the colon from a cystic lesion. This is particularly valuable in evaluating incidental pararenal cystic areas not visible by radiographic methods.

LXP — SERIES

The line between the xiphoid process and symphysis pubis in normal individuals also crosses the umbilicus and is called the *LXP line.* The LXP plane transecting the midportion of the body is designated as LXP−0 and all the sections toward the patient's right side are LXP plus (LXP+1, +2, +3) while sections toward the patient's left side are LXP minus (LXP−1, −2, −3).

FIGURE 1.19
Supine longitudinal scan. The fluid-filled colon may simulate a cystic mass. An echo-free tubular structure is situated above the psoas muscle. The configuration may change with peristalsis, which is best documented on the A-scope. Serial scans may demonstrate that the right or left colon merges with the fluid-filled transverse colon. Fluid filled colon from acute peritonitis. Head is toward the right.

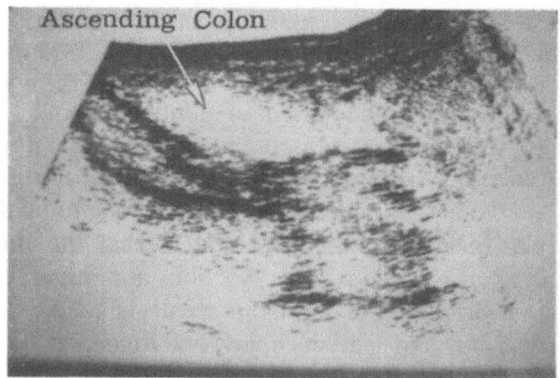

POSTERIOR PROJECTION

PTC — SERIES

In the posterior projection the transcrestal line or plane represents the zero point and is called the *PTC* (Posterior Transcrestal Plane). The transcrestal plane is PTC–0 and all sections above this plane are PTC plus (PTC+1, +2, +3).

PLS — SERIES

The spine is in the reference point for posterior views and sections, *PLS* (Posterior Longitudinal Spine). Toward the right side are PLS plus sections (PLS +1, +2, +3), and to the left are PLS minus sections (PLS −1, −2, −3).

DECUBITUS PROJECTION

TRANSVERSE DECUBITUS

In the lateral projection, with the patient lying on his side, the crest of the ilium is the zero point and all planes above it are plus cuts. If the patient's right side is up, he is said to be lying in the right lateral decubitus (RDC) position and if his left side is up, he is in the left lateral decubitus (LDC) position (Right Decubitus Crest or Left Decubitus Crest). The word *decubitus* in ultrasound refers to the side of the examination closest to the sonic beam. Sections above the crest ilium are LDC – plus (LDC = Plane (LDC–0) LDC+1, +2, +3; RDC = Plane RDC +1, +2, +3).

LONGITUDINAL DECUBITUS

In longitudinal sections the axillary line becomes the reference point. Therefore, all sections anterior to the right (RDA) or left (LDA) decubitus axillary line are plus sections (RDA+1, +2, and LDA+1, +2) and sections posterior to the axillary lines are minus sections (RDA−1, −2, and LDA−1, −2).

ERECT PROJECTION

If the patient is sitting, instead of the word decubitus (D) we use the word *erect* (E) and ab-

breviations such as REC or LEC, and REA or LEA. These views are specifically used to study the chest wall, as for pleural effusion, and to evaluate the effect of gravity on abdominal structures, ptotic organ, or positional changes of organ relationships in normal and abnormal conditions in the supine, semierect, and erect positions.

ANGULATION

If the transducer is pointing toward the head or the right side, the degree of angulation relative to the perpendicular body section is designated plus. Toward the feet or toward the left side it is minus. For example, ATC+2+15° is the section 2 cm above the transcrestal line in anterior projection with a 15° angulation toward the head.

SUBCOSTAL AND INTERCOSTAL SECTIONS

Subcostal sectional study starts at the xiphoid and runs parallel to the ribs from the xiphoid process. Intercostal section is similar to subcostal. On the right side it is RSC, and on the left side it is LSC. The rib itself is the zero point. Thus RSC–0 is meaningless because the rib produces a sonic shadow. The section below the pertinent rib will be numbered accordingly. For example, RSC−11 is a section below the 11th rib on the right side and LSC-11 is the section above the 11th rib on the left side.

TRANSDUCER CONTACT

Various scanning planes are utilized during a routine study. If the plane of interest does not lie perpendicular to the body surface, acoustic contact may be impaired. As a result a large number of echoes are lost during scanning if sectional planes are perpendicular to the table rather than to the patient. To prevent loss of contact at curved areas of the body, the examiner must direct the transducer perpendicular to the body contour to achieve maximum beam intensity.

SENSITIVITY SETTING OR ATTENUATION

As in routine ECG tracings, the sonographer should establish a standard baseline sensitivity setting for each organ to avoid confusion in interpretation. After each study or section, the attenuation may be changed to differentiate various components of an organ or cystic from solid masses.

The frequency of ultrasound determines the average attenuation beam pattern (20). Using a higher frequency and a shorter sonic pulse, a narrower beam may be obtained, which increases resolution. By lowering the frequency, deep structures can be visualized better. At higher frequency, deep structures reflect weak echoes (20). These produce serious problems in diagnosis, and can be corrected by adjusting the time gain compensation (TGC) control. The TGC corrects for higher average absorption (37). This adjustment must be made when an organ returns echoes at a certain frequency but does not return them at another frequency. In this case the pattern of the beam from the transducer has changed or the receiver is not properly compensating for average attenuation loss.

GAIN SETTING OR TGC CHANGE DURING STUDY

Opinion varies regarding changing TGC settings during scanning. One group is in favor of changing the TGC during the study, if it is necessary (36), because the attenuation of sonic waves varies in different organs. Consequently, it is difficult to outline the entire organ in one plane, with a fixed attenuation. On the other hand, changing the attenuation control during the examination may produce artifacts. These problems are avoided with gray-scale systems.

FACTORS ALTERING NORMAL ACOUSTIC IMAGE

There are certain limitations to, and problems inherent in, each study. Some can easily be avoided; others, which are extremely difficult to prevent, are:

1. Respiratory motion.
2. Marked dehydration can be avoided by proper hydration.
3. Gas in the bowel. Gas interferes with sound transmission and the deep abdominal and retroperitoneal regions cannot be properly evaluated. Therefore, the study should be repeated after the patient has been given a laxative and a cleansing enema. When excessive gas is in the stomach, the semi-erect position allows the gas to rise to the fundus where it will not interfere with the scan of abdominal organs. As previously described, bone effectively blocks the ultrasonic beam and no information is gained distal to a bony structure.
4. Presence of radiographic contrast in the gastrointestinal tract. Water-soluble contrast material in the gastrointestinal tract does not alter gross anatomy nor the transmission of ultrasonic waves through the abdominal contents. With barium in the gastrointestinal tract, even with high-gain setting only the anterior aspect of the bowel is detectable for imaging (50). Barium blocks the passage of ultrasound to organs located behind barium-filled loops of bowel. This problem can be detected by a plain film of the abdomen and a history of contrast examination.
5. Deep mediastinal area and lung pathology cannot be evaluated by sonography because the air-containing lung transmits ultrasound poorly.
6. The pelvic bone prevents evaluation of structures deep in the pelvic cavity. Evaluation of this area can be improved by using an internal transducer.
7. Resolution of systems. At the present time, commercially available units have limited resolution, and deep intra-abdominal structures, smaller than 1 cm, cannot be evaluated by conventional presentation or gray scale.

TOPOGRAPHIC MARKING OF SUSPICIOUS AREA

In any ultrasound department, a water-soluble dye or grease pencil should be available so that an organ or area of interest can be marked upon the skin. Multiple markings of suspected pathology will allow this area to be scanned in the plane marked off on the skin. If the area is constant in this plane and also demonstrated in a perpendicular plane, then it is a true area of disease as opposed to an artefact (34).

ORIENTATION OF SCAN

The sonographer can find the true orientation of an organ or area of pathology by making appropriate markings on the skin and scanning in this plane. Three-dimensional visualization is obtained when the area perpendicular to the markings is scanned.

MARKING THE BODY WITH THE TRANSDUCER

By convention, the symphysis pubis is marked with an angle and the umbilicus or transcrestal plane is designated by a perpendicular line.

MARKING THE POLAROID PICTURE

For complete information (as in x-ray techniques) each polaroid picture should have at least two figures on the front. The first figure represents distance from reference points (either transversely or longitudinally) in centimeters. The second is used to show the gain setting, sensitivity setting, or attenuation. A third number may be used to designate the angle of tilt. The name, date, age, and sex of the patient will appear on the back of the polaroid picture, or these data may be digitized on to the scan by a computer. After each polaroid is labeled, it is good practice to string each in sequence on a strip of masking tape.

VISUAL ORIENTATION OF POLAROID PRINTS

Anterior abdominal transverse scans are viewed from below. Longitudinal scans are viewed from the left side of the patient in the supine, and from the right side of the patient in the prone position.

SIMULTANEOUS DISPLAY OF A-MODE WITH B-SCAN

During the course of B-scanning, any anechoic or echo-free area can be verified by A-mode. For example, the aorta is detected and identified by a narrow echo-free area between two high spikes that exhibit a characteristic "to-and-fro" motion on the A-scope.

Because of the nature of the electronic threshold of the B-scan, an echo of low intensity will not be registered; hence a mass with few internal echoes may be considered cystic in the B-scan. On the other hand, the small internal echoes displayed on the A-scope greatly add to diagnostic accuracy. Also, echo artefacts of gas and bone as well as the "loud echo" artefact from a relatively sonolucent area can be observed on the A-scope and corrected.

DETECTION OF THROUGH TRANSMISSION PATTERN

Through transmission is the sound energy that passes through a structure and is then recorded by the receiving transducer. It is inversely proportional to the attenuating properties of the medium and is registered on the oscilloscope as the number of echoes and their amplitude at the distal interface of the region insonated.

To evaluate transmission characteristics of a structure, the posterior border of that structure must be identified. The distal border is visualized at low-sensitivity settings when the medium is highly transonic, as in fluid structures and parenchymatous glands, such as the liver and spleen. When the medium is poorly transonic, the sound beam is attenuated significantly and sensitivity must be increased to amplify distal echoes. This is particularly true for solid, acoustically homogeneous tumors, such as leiomyomata and lymphomas. Indeed, maximum-gain settings may be necessary to faintly image the distal wall. These masses may not contain sufficient internal interfaces to produce echoes and may appear as sonolucent lesions. In these cases, the echo-free region is differentiated from a cyst by a poorly delineated posterior wall, indicating poor through transmission (Fig. 1.20).

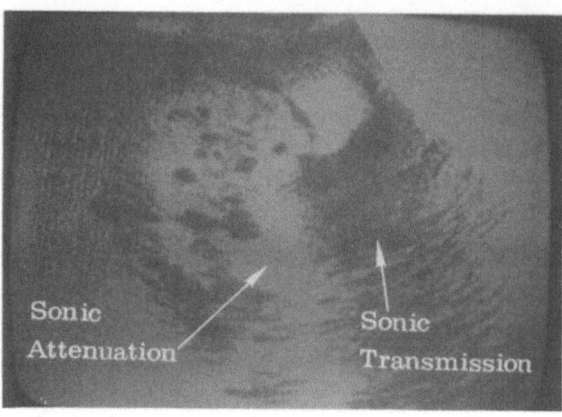

FIGURE 1.20
Through transmission. In above gray-scale study, note the through transmission pattern posterior to the fluid content structure and attenuation of sonic beam in solid architecture.

Through transmission does not occur when scanning over bone, barium, or air. Air interfaces reflect, bony interfaces absorb, and heavy metals tend to scatter sound. The net effect is a lack of penetration of the ultrasonic beam. During the scan, a sonic shadow is noted when the transducer is passed over bone, barium, or air. If the incident sonic energy is sufficient, reflection artefacts may be noted over air and bone. The artefacts appear as a series of echoes spaced at equal intervals, gradually diminishing in amplitude. These electronic artefacts must not be confused with echoes from deep interfaces.

Sonic shadowing is best appreciated during linear scanning with B-mode and by simultaneously noting abrupt termination of A-scope echoes in a single high amplitude echo. During compound scanning, the posterior border of an ultrasonically shadowed region may be filled-in with echoes, spuriously creating a distal interface. The examiner must exercise great caution when scanning over bone or bowel so as not to "create" an echo-free lesion.

Tumors with internal degeneration permit better through transmission than do architecturally intact masses of the same histologic type (51). Production of fluid-filled necrotic spaces within a tumor increases beam transmission and ap-

pears on the oscilloscope as a lesion with multiple posterior echoes. At low sensitivity, anterior and posterior borders of a degenerating tumor may be outlined and the high posterior echo density may simulate a simple cyst. This error is avoided by sensitivity studies in which a characteristic echogenic mass is revealed as gain is increased. Indeed, certain tumors have a biologic tendency to degenerate (leiomyomas, liposarcomas, renal cell carcinomas), and by demonstrating increased through transmission in a previously poorly transmitting tumor internal degeneration can be documented, which may aid in histosonographic tissue typing.

A highly transonic structure may exhibit a low posterior echo density when the distal interface lies adjacent to bone or air. Known as a reverse sonic shadow, this occurs when a lesion's distal wall lies next to a gas-containing viscus (a renal cyst whose posterior wall lies over the air-filled colon) or bony surface (pancreatic pseudocyst lying over the spine). The presence of a sharply outlined distal wall will alert the sonographer to the possibility of such acoustic damping and the area should be rescanned in multiple projections to demonstrate the intrinsic, high through transmission of the transonic structure (Fig. 1.20).

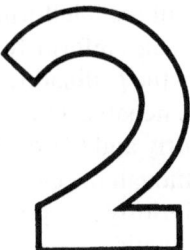

hepatic sonography

GENERAL INTRODUCTION

The liver was initially studied by the water bath technique (41). Since then, contact, compound scanning techniques have given echotomographic studies of diagnostic quality in hepatic disorders.

Sonography is unique in that it can localize an intrahepatic lesion and assess its nature. The final diagnosis can be established through ultrasonically guided cyst puncture and cytologic study of the aspirate.

Ultrasonic examination for a space-occupying lesion of the liver is complimentary to isotopic scanning and to angiography. However, it is superior to other methods for guiding a needle through the liver to sample a lesion.

THE LIVER

ANATOMY

The liver occupies the right hypochondrium and may normally extend to the left lateral chest wall. The outer

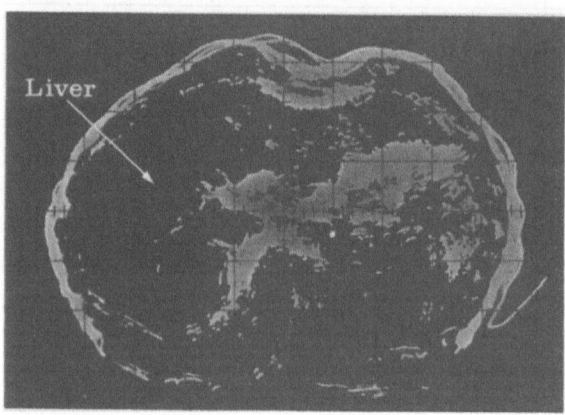

FIGURE 2.1
Supine transverse scan. B-mode at low sensitivity. At low-gain settings, homogeneous liver tissue appears echo-free since low-level echoes are not displayed on the oscilloscope.

FIGURE 2.2
Supine transverse scan. At higher sensitivity, the liver parenchyma fills-in with echoes. Note right kidney below the hepatic substance.

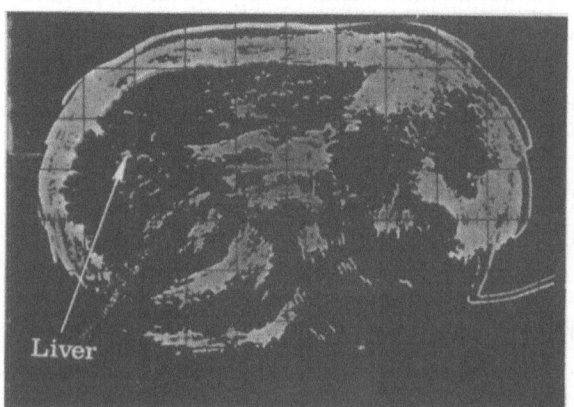

surface is rounded, and the liver is divided into a large right and a smaller left lobe. This partition occurs in the plane of the falciform ligament. The quadrate lobe lies inferiorly and is bounded on the right by the gallbladder and posteriorly by the porta hepatis. The caudate lobe is situated posteriorly and lies cephalad to the porta hepatis, although the caudate process may extend inferiorly to a position posterior to the porta hepatis.

Superior, is the dome of the right diaphragm and a portion of the left diaphragm. Anterior, are the diaphragm and the 6th to 10th anterior ribs. On the right, the upper two-thirds lies in contact with the diaphragm and lung base. The lower lateral one-third is adjacent to the chest wall. The visceral surface of the liver has grooves for the right colon, right kidney, duodenum, gallbladder, porta hepatis, and inferior vena cava.

The liver is largely intraperitoneal and is surrounded by a connective tissue capsule. The hepatic veins empty into the inferior vena cava, which may pass through the dorsal aspect of the liver. The portal vein and hepatic artery enter the gland through the porta hepatis and branch throughout the liver pulp. The biliary tree empties the liver through the common hepatic duct, passing in the porta hepatis.

SONOANATOMY

Since the normal liver is postioned almost entirely beneath the ribs, ultrasonic scanning is technically difficult due to sonic attenuation and reverberation artifacts caused by the rib cage.

At low sensitivity, the liver appears as an echo-free organ (Fig. 2.1) with a concave distal border overlying the gallbladder, inferior vena cava, aorta, and pancreas. At higher gain settings, the liver fills with echoes (Fig. 2.2). These weak echoes, shaped like dots or short lines, are reflections from larger biliary radicles and hepatic vessels. Using the gray scale, the liver is more echogenic than the kidney (Fig. 2.3a and b) or spleen and less echogenic than the pancreas.

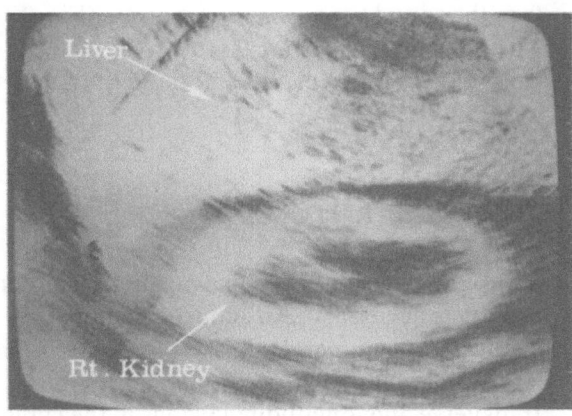

FIGURE 2-3 (a)

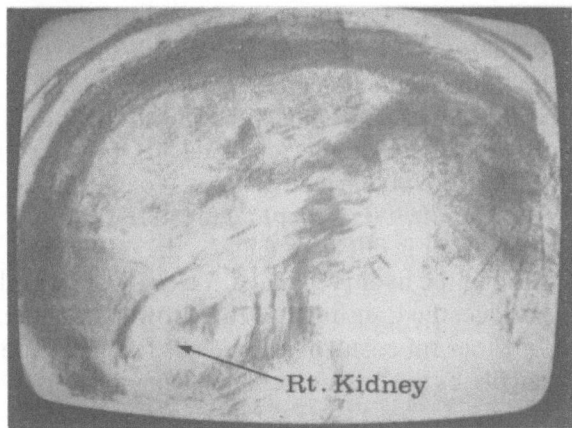

FIGURE 2-3 (b)

FIGURE 2-4

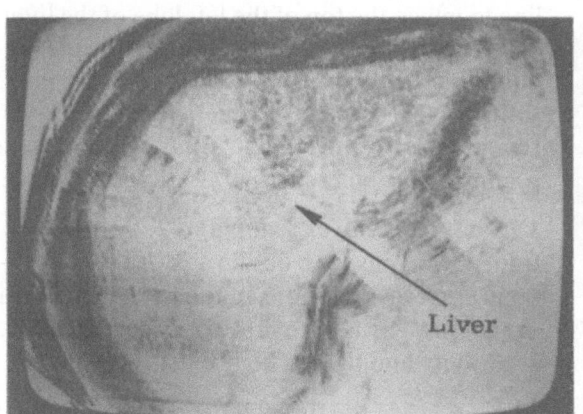

In transverse section, the liver fills the right upper quadrant and crosses the midline, as the left lobe, for a varying distance (Fig. 2.4). Beneath the concave capsular echo pattern from the liver are the echoes from the right kidney, an echo-free inferior vena cava, and the aorta. The medium gray echoes of the liver are seen above the light gray renal parenchyma and dark gray collecting system of the right kidney. The aorta and inferior vena cava are echo free (Fig. 2.5).

In longitudinal section, various structures may be identified below the liver, such as the aorta, pancreas, and antrum of the stomach immediately beneath the inferior margin of the liver. The dome of the liver and right diaphragm are noted as a concave, high-amplitude echo sur-

FIGURE 2.3 (a)
Supine longitudinal scan. The homogeneous liver parenchyma is more echogenic than the renal parenchyma.

FIGURE 2.3 (b)
Supine transverse scan. Note the medium-gray echo texture of the normal liver substance in contrast to the light-gray echoes of the renal cortex and dark-gray echoes of the renal collecting system.

FIGURE 2.4
Supine transverse scan. The left lobe of the normal liver may lie in the left upper quadrant. Note the homogeneous internal architecture of low-amplitude echoes.

FIGURE 2.5
Supine transverse scan. Regional anatomy of the liver. The hepatic substance is more echogenic than the renal cortex. The aorta and inferior vena cava are the echo-free rounded structures anterior to the spine.

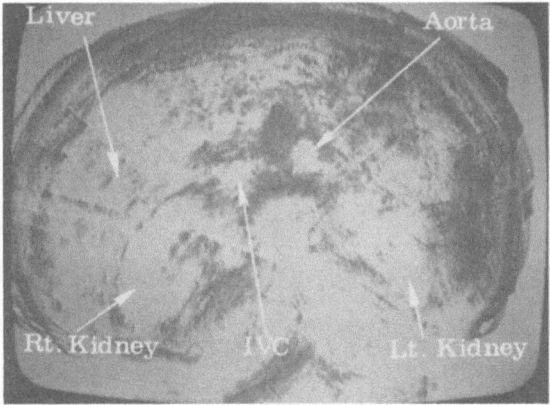

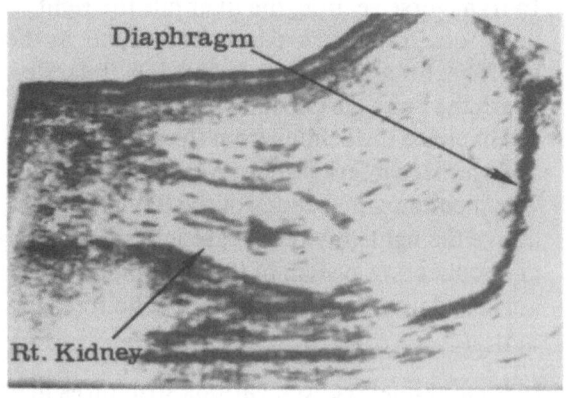

FIGURE 2.6
Supine longitudinal scan. The right diaphragm appears as a highly echogenic arc. Sound is not transmitted beyond the diaphragm. Head is toward the right.

FIGURE 2.7
Right lateral decubitus scan. The liver may be scanned in the decubitus position. This permits good visualization of the posterior liver parenchyma and the relationship of the liver to the right kidney. Intercostal scanning is easier in the decubitus position.

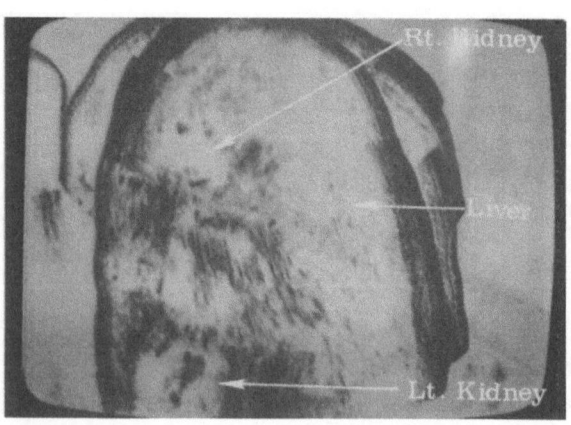

face the sound beam cannot penetrate (Fig. 2.6). The inferior vena cava passes through the dorsal aspect of the liver and empties into the right atrium.

SONOLAPAROTOMY

The patient lies in the supine position. No preparation is necessary. An acoustic coupling agent, such as mineral oil, is applied to the skin. The usual scanning procedure employs the transverse and longitudinal planes in the supine position. When the oblique intercostal and oblique subcostal planes (Fig. 2.7) are scanned, the patient lies supine or left side down.

Transverse scanning starts from the lower border of the visualized hepatic substance and continues to the liver—lung interface. Some examiners start from the midthorax and scan downwards. Sections are made at 1-cm intervals, with varying gain settings. To image the dome of the liver—diaphragm interface, the transducer is tilted cranially as the upper one-third of the liver is scanned. To see the visceral surface, the transducer is tilted toward the feet. In either subcostal or intercostal scanning, one angulates the transducer approximately 10° to 15°.

Longitudinal scanning planes pass through the spine, and this fixed structure is used as the axis of transducer rotation. Longitudinal sections are performed from the right midaxillary line (transducer parallel to the table), with rotational intervals of 10° towards the left midclavicular line to image the top of the left lobe of the liver. The dome of the liver is best shown during longitudinal sectioning, when the transducer is gently pressed under the liver edge and sector scanning performed (Fig. 2.6). As in transverse scanning, various sensitivity settings are used.

During routine liver scanning a 2.25-MHz transducer is used to obtain a series of longitudinal and cross-sections of the liver and regional anatomy. Scans are first performed at low sensitivity and then at high sensitivity.

The outline of the three dimensions of the liver

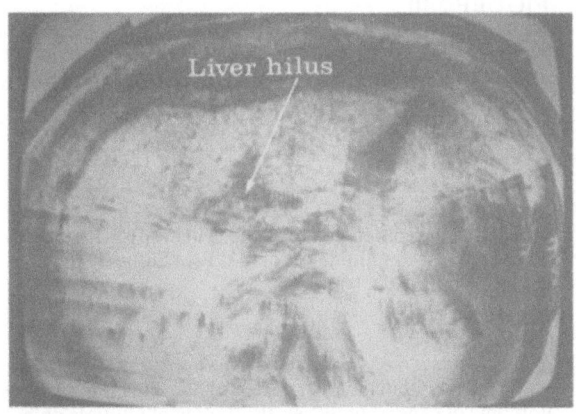

FIGURE 2-8

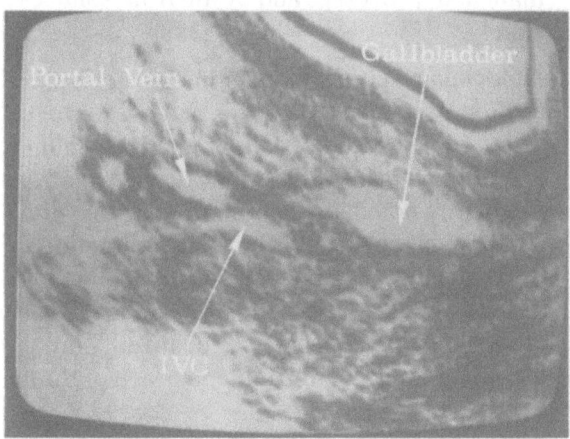

FIGURE 2-9 (a)

FIGURE 2-9 (b)

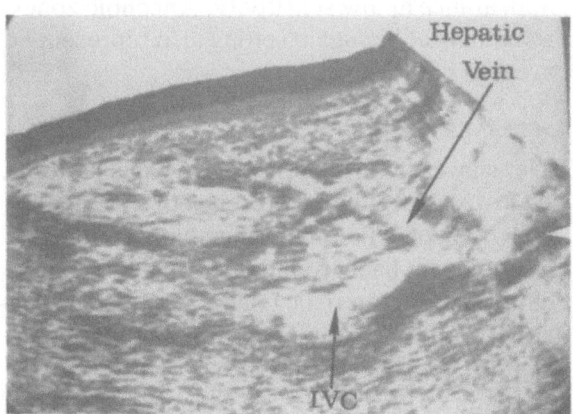

provides an estimate of liver volume. The procedure is done at low sensitivity to highlight alterations in liver parenchyma caused by acoustic impedance.

The liver is sonographically homogeneous during B-scanning. An exception is its hilum, where major blood vessels and ducts provide an acoustically inhomogeneous interface. At low sensitivity, the liver is echo free except for its outer boundaries and hilus. As sensitivity is increased, the gland fills-in with echoes and becomes an homogeneous collection of dots on the B-scan image.

The increased resolution noted with scan converters shows the normal liver homogeneously filled with gray echoes, throughout which are scattered multiple, linear, echo-free areas with dark gray walls projecting toward the hilum. These most likely represent major portal and hepatic venous structures (Fig. 2.8).

The porta hepatis may be localized with grayscale and real-time scanners by imaging the common bile duct (if enlarged) or portal vein. These appear as echo-free tubular structures (79) (Fig. 2.9a). The hepatic veins empty into the inferior vena cava (Fig. 2.9b).

SONOPATHOLOGY

Locating pathology by sonotomograms is relatively easy. However, it may be quite difficult to determine the nature of the lesion. Diagnostic criteria aid in differentiating benign from

FIGURE 2.8
Supine transverse scan. Echo-free tubular structures point toward the hilum of the liver. This normal echo pattern represents the hilar vessels.

FIGURE 2.9 (a)
Supine longitudinal scan. The porta hepatis is localized by following the portal vein into the liver. The inferior vena cava dorsal to the portal vein.

FIGURE 2.9 (b)
Supine longitudinal scan. The inferior vena cava ascends into the right atrium. Before it passes through the diaphragm it usually receives a branch of the hepatic vein. Head is toward the right.

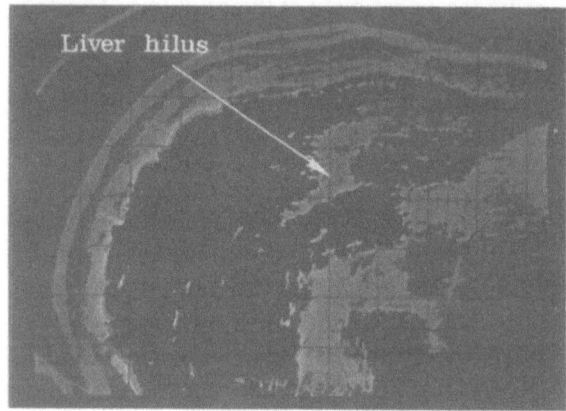

FIGURE 2-10

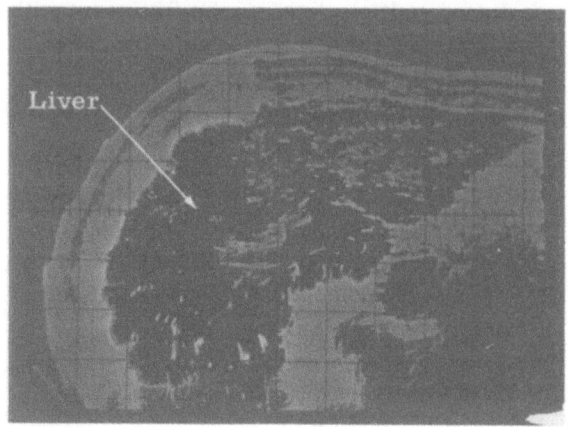

FIGURE 2-11

FIGURE 2-12

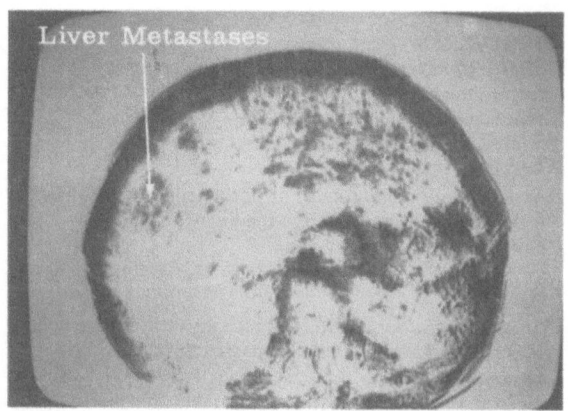

FIGURE 2.10
Supine transverse scan. B-mode at medium sensitivity. The branching echo pattern of the normal liver hilus may appear either as a transverse medially extending band of echoes or as an echogenic septum in the anteroposterior plane of the midportion of the liver.

FIGURE 2.11
Supine transverse scan. Discrete separate echoes appear within the liver parenchyma as the sensitivity is increased. These are low-amplitude echoes and are diffusely noted throughout the liver.

FIGURE 2.12
Supine transverse scan. Typical ring appearance of metastatic focus within the liver parenchyma. This is not pathognomonic of cancer; however, the finding of multiple defects is highly suggestive of liver metastases.

malignant processes and cystic from solid lesions.

At low-gain setting, two distinctive echo patterns may be noted in the normal liver. Most often, a linear band of echoes from the hilum extends in a medial direction (Fig. 2.10). Less frequently noted is a septum transversing the parenchyma in an anteroposterior direction in the region of the hilum. The normal hilum is located at the junction of the right and left lobes of the liver and appears as a localized, branching echo pattern on the under surface of the liver.

As stated, by increasing gain setting, the echo-free normal liver parenchyma changes its pattern and numerous, clearly separated weak echoes are displayed (Fig. 2.11). Abnormal weak echoes accumulate in one location, with a circumscribed homogeneous pattern or a ring appearance at low sensitivity. Anechoic zones remaining at high-gain setting also represent areas of pathology.

METASTASES

Metastases in the liver have two basic patterns. At low sensitivity, the presence of a round collection of echoes or a ring-shaped pattern in a sonolucent background of normal liver parenchyma is characteristic (Fig. 2.12). At high sensitivity, areas of sonolucency in diffusely echogenic hepatic tissues are the second typical appearance (37) (Fig. 2.13). Any abnormality in

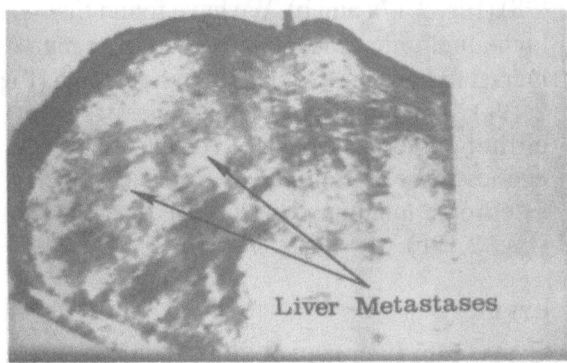

FIGURE 2-13

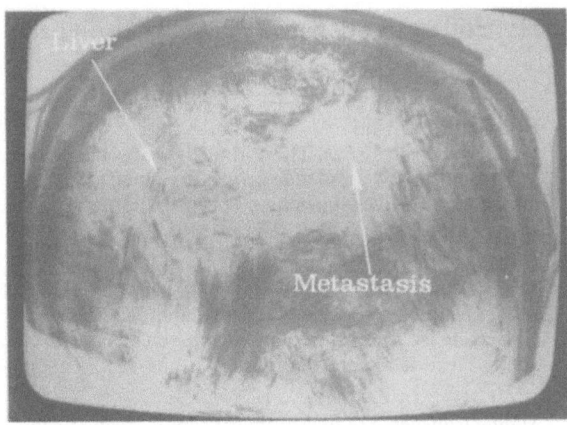

FIGURE 2-14

FIGURE 2-15

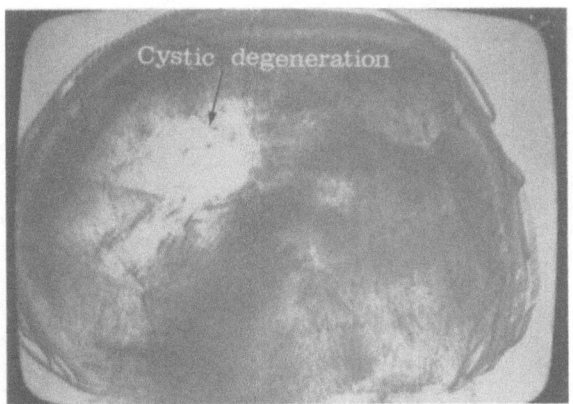

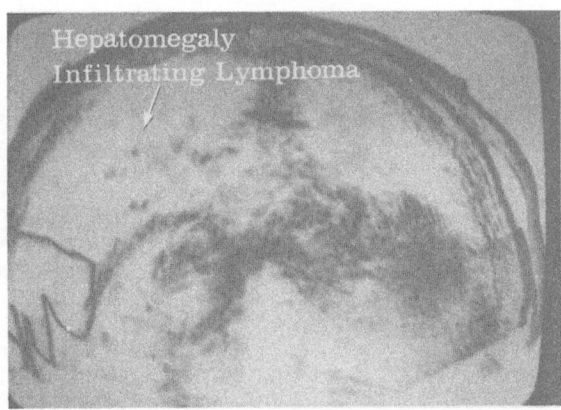

echographic anatomy must be documented in both longitudinal and cross-section.

A different pattern occurs when the liver is almost completely replaced by metastatic tumor (Fig. 2.14), or by an infiltrating tumor, such as lymphoma. In massive metastases with necrosis the liver appears cystic, with irregular borders (Fig. 2.15). Substitution of liver parenchyma by tumor may produce an acoustically homogeneous medium that strongly attenuates sound energy. The liver appears echo free at medium and high sensitivities and the posterior wall is poorly defined (Fig. 2.16).

It has been stated that the most common appearance of metastases on gray scale is that of low-amplitude echoes within the higher amplitude echoes of the normal hepatic substance

FIGURE 2.13
Supine transverse scan. Note multiple anechoic regions within the liver parenchyma at high sensitivity. Sonolucent areas represent foci of necrotic metastatic adenocarcinoma.

FIGURE 2.14
Supine transverse scan. Huge sonolucent zone with high through transmission. This cystic appearing region represents a massive region of tumor replacement in the liver. Note the irregular distal wall.

FIGURE 2.15
Supine transverse scan. Cystic appearance of huge metastatic area occupying most of the liver substance. Echo-free area has irregular distal wall.

FIGURE 2.16
Supine transverse scan. The liver is diffusely infiltrated with lymphoma. This liver parenchyma appears echo poor and the tumor markedly attenuates the sound so that the adjacent right kidney is poorly imaged.

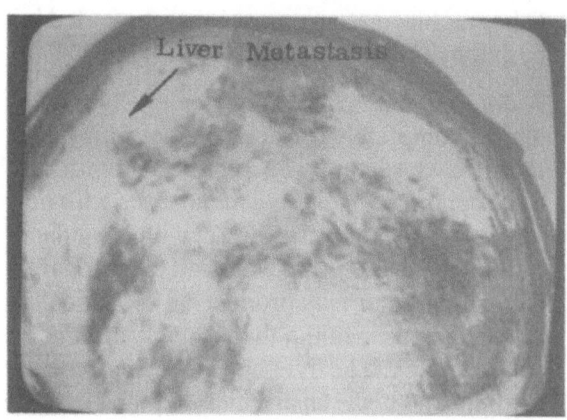

FIGURE 2-17 (a)

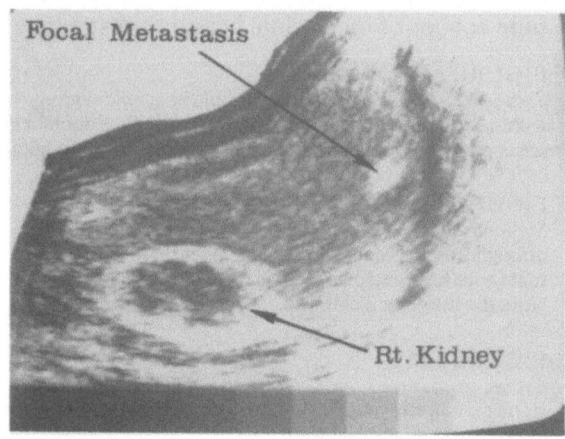

FIGURE 2-17 (b)

FIGURE 2-18

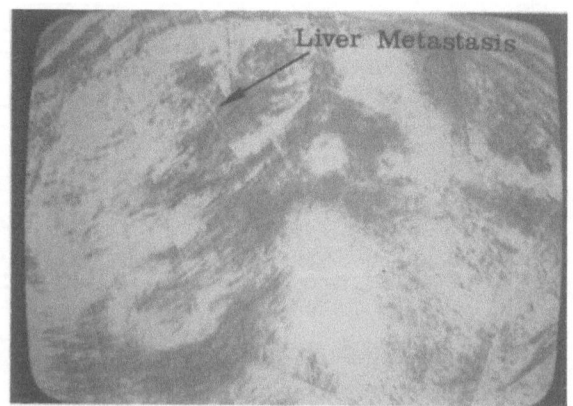

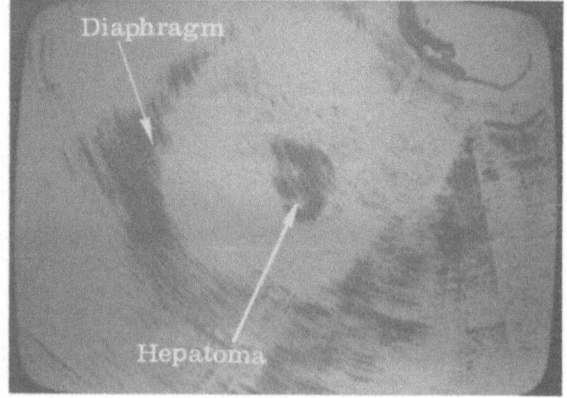

(78) (Fig. 2.17a and b). We have found that high-amplitude echoes more often represent metastatic disease (Fig. 2.18) or hepatoma (Fig. 2.19a). The majority of hepatomas occur in cirrhotic livers. Multiple, irregular, thick echoes represent diffuse liver disease, such as chronic inflammatory disease or metastases (Fig. 2.19b).

CYSTS

Cysts of the liver may be congenital. These are usually small and associated with polycystic changes in other organs, such as the kidney. If the cysts are larger than 1.5 cm, they will be detected as echo-free areas on gray-scale systems (Fig. 2.20a and b).

Hydatid cysts are usually large when detected;

FIGURE 2.17 (a)
Supine transverse scan. The normal liver appears echogenic. Regions of low-amplitude echoes are noted scattered throughout the liver substance. This is the common appearance of metastatic adenocarcinoma.

FIGURE 2.17 (b)
Supine longitudinal scan. A well defined low level zone of echoes is noted just below the right diaphragm. This was not seen in isotope scan; follow-up proved metastatic carcinoma. Head is toward the right.

FIGURE 2.18
Supine transverse scan. Multiple discrete irregular echogenic foci are present within the liver. This is a frequent pattern of metastatic carcinoma.

FIGURE 2.19 (a)
Supine longitudinal scan. Note cluster of high-amplitude echoes in the center of the liver. This might represent a metastatic focus but proved to be a hepatoma in a non-cirrhotic liver.

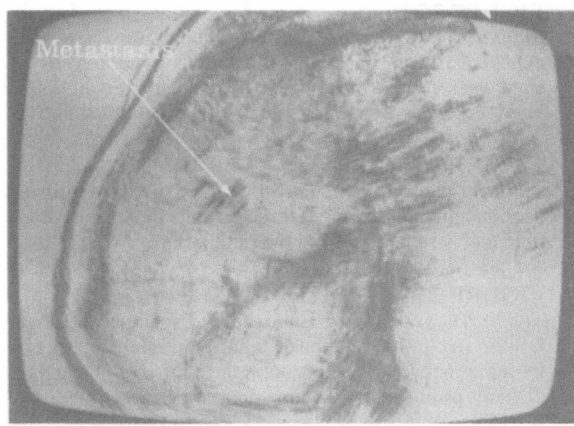

FIGURE 2-19 (b)

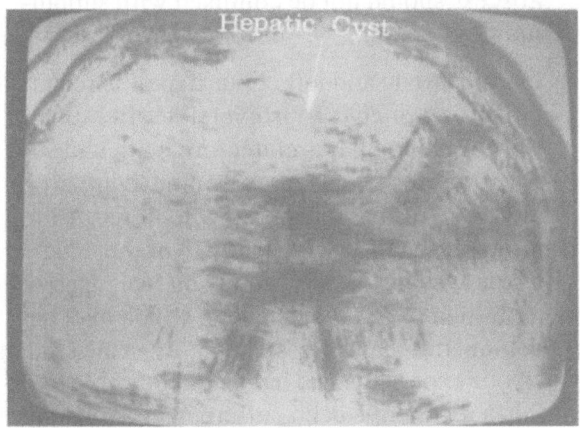

FIGURE 2-20 (a)

FIGURE 2-20 (b)

the simple echinococcal cyst appears echo free. Often septae, necrotic debris, and internal cysts produce the picture of an echogenic mass. Occasionally a ring-like pattern within a cyst may be observed and indicates a daughter cyst. This inflammatory appearance is highly specific for hydatid disease (44).

INFLAMMATORY PROCESSES

Inflammatory conditions of the liver include infectious and toxic disorders. Abscess formation may be pyogenic and appear as single or multiple, irregular, echo-free areas within the hepatic parenchyma (Fig. 2.21). An amebic abscess is usually located in the posterior portion of the right lobe of the liver. It appears as a complex mass with irregular walls and a high degree of through transmission. Liver abscesses regress more rapidly by ultrasound than by

FIGURE 2.19 (b)
Supine transverse scan. Multiple thick irregular echoes are demonstrated throughout the liver. This pattern may represent chronic inflammatory changes or metastatic carcinoma. Metastatic adenocarcinoma.

FIGURE 2.20 (a)
Supine transverse scan. Echo-free zone within the left lobe of the liver, with an oblique septum. Congenital cyst of the liver. Note high through transmission distal to the cyst.

FIGURE 2.20 (b)
Supine longitudinal scan. Anechoic cyst with incomplete septal echoes and sharply outlined distal wall. Note expansion of liver outline.

FIGURE 2.21
Supine transverse scan. B-mode at high sensitivity reveals an echo-free region with irregular margins in the right lobe of the liver. Abscess of the liver.

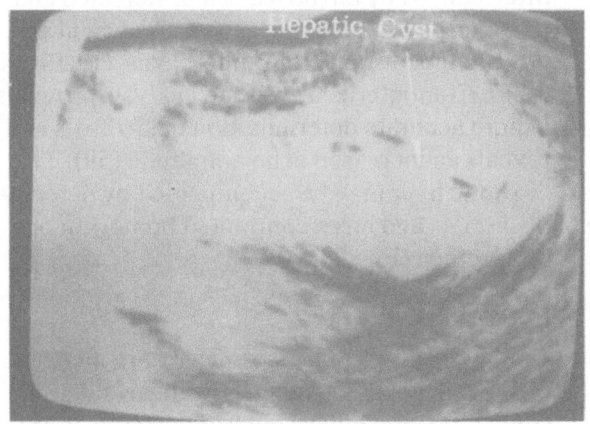

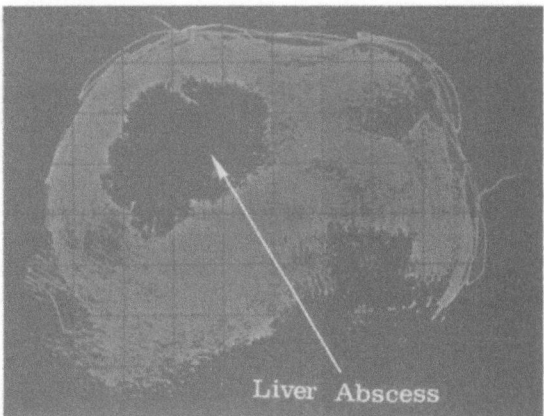

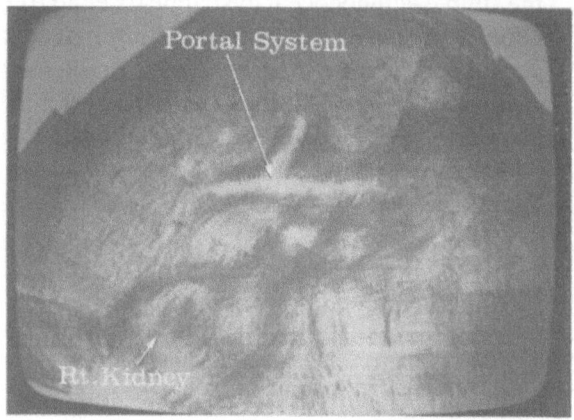

FIGURE 2-22

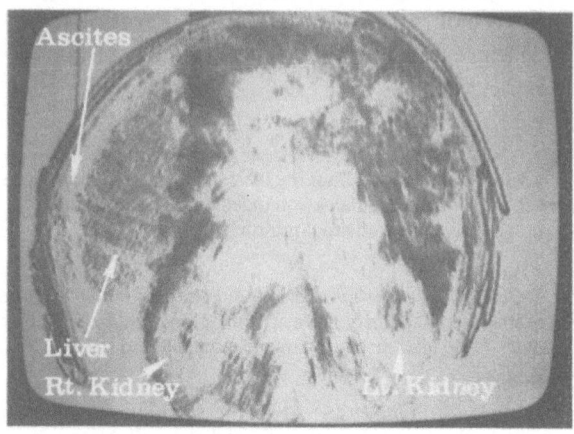

FIGURE 2-23

FIGURE 2-24

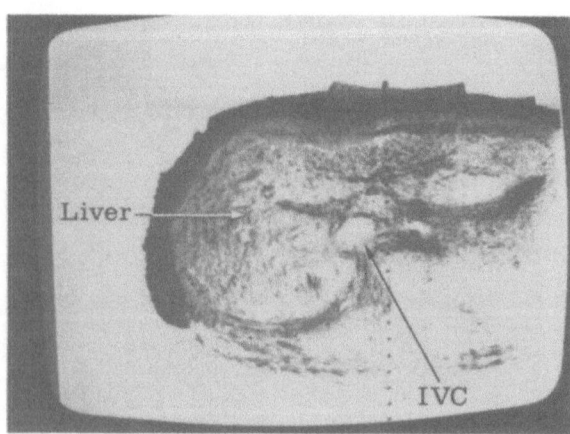

FIGURE 2.22
Supine transverse scan. The liver echo pattern is more echogenic than usual. There is a paucity of echo-free small vessels. The portal vein and its main branches are dilated. Portal hypertension due to cirrhosis of the liver.

FIGURE 2.23
Supine transverse scan. Cirrhosis of the liver is frequently accompanied by ascites. The liver floats in the echo-free fluid and is separated from the right kidney.

FIGURE 2.24
Supine transverse scan. Enlarged liver in congestive heart failure. In chronic right heart failure the echogenicity of the liver parenchyma depends upon the degree of fibrotic changes produced by the long-standing heart failure.

isotopic scanning. Perihepatic abscesses are noted as irregular anechoic regions in the subphrenic and subhepatic spaces. A subphrenic abscess should not be confused with subpulmonic effusion.

Chronic toxic and infectious hepatitis results in cirrhosis, which is an irreversible alteration of the normal lobular architecture, with widespread fibrosis replacing atrophic liver parenchyma. Areas of regenerating liver tissue are interspersed diffusely. The size of the liver varies; however, there is usually an increased echo pattern in the liver substance, which may be demonstrated on B-scan and gray-scale studies. In our experience we have not been able to obtain a distinctive echo pattern in cirrhotic patients. This may be due to the wide spectrum of changes caused by fatty metamorphosis, connective tissue proliferation, regenerating nodules, and necrosis in various combination. However, portal hypertension, which is most often caused by cirrhosis, can be detected and presents as a dilated portal venous system and an absence of smaller peripheral vessels (Fig. 2.22). Computerized A-mode analysis provides a more accurate determination of cirrhosis and reveals an increased echo amplitude (59). The cirrhotic liver may be accompanied by detectable ascites and has a contracted homogeneous appearance (Fig. 2.23).

HEPATOMEGALY

Common causes of hepatomegaly are metastatic disease, hepatitis, congestive heart failure (Fig. 2.24), and biliary obstruction (Fig. 2.25).

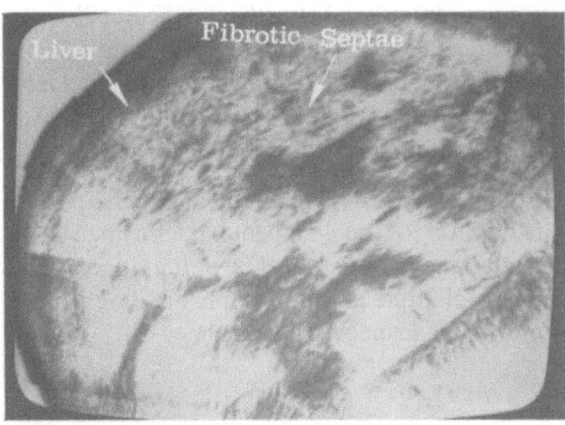

FIGURE 2-25 (a)

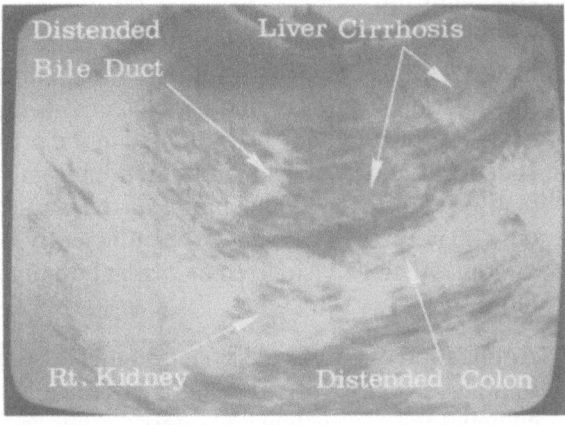

FIGURE 2-25 (b)

FIGURE 2.26
Supine longitudinal scan. Riedel's lobe is a normal variation of the right lobe of the liver. This right lobe extends into the right pelvis and may be mistaken for hepatomegaly or a mass lesion.

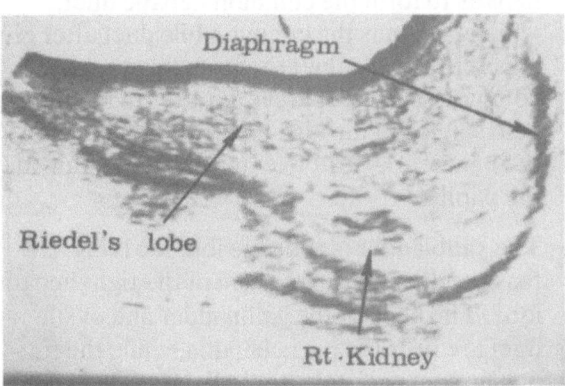

FIGURE 2.25 (a)
Supine transverse scan. Hepatomegaly from long-standing biliary obstructión. Echogenic pattern of liver stroma due to fibrosis produced by biliary cirrhosis.

FIGURE 2.25 (b)
Supine longitudinal scan. The liver is echogenic and dilatation of the intrahepatic biliary ducts is demonstrated. Dorsal to the liver is the right kidney. Caudal to the kidney is a segment of dilated ascending colon. Carcinoma of colon with metastatic nodes in the porta hepatis. Dilated colon is due to distal obstruction.

However, the liver may be palpable without coexistent hepatomegaly. Emphysema and asthma, with low diaphragms or aberrant lobes such as Riedel's lobe, are examples (Fig. 2.26). The liver may be enlarged but not palpable in cirrhosis, posterior enlargement, and marked obesity.

VOLUME DETERMINATION

Ultrasonic scanning gives a three-dimensional representation of the liver, which allows a rough estimate of volume. Computerized analysis of ultrasonic sections permits an accurate determination of liver volume (66).

GUIDED PUNCTURE BIOPSY

The percutaneous puncture transducer now enables the clinician to needle lesions with great accuracy and to aspirate their contents. This transducer has a special central bore through which puncture needles of various sizes can be passed. The fine-gauge needle produces minimal trauma to tissues.

When an echogenic zone, at low sensitivity, or a sonolucent region, at high sensitivity, is delineated, percutaneous cyst puncture may be performed with minimal patient preparation. Coagulopathy should be ruled out by history and laboratory determinations. The skin is sterilized and draped. The scanning transducer is then replaced with a sterile puncture transducer. The sound beam is directed into the zone of interest, and the depth of the lesion from the skin surface is readily measured from the echo pattern on the calibrated A-mode oscilloscope

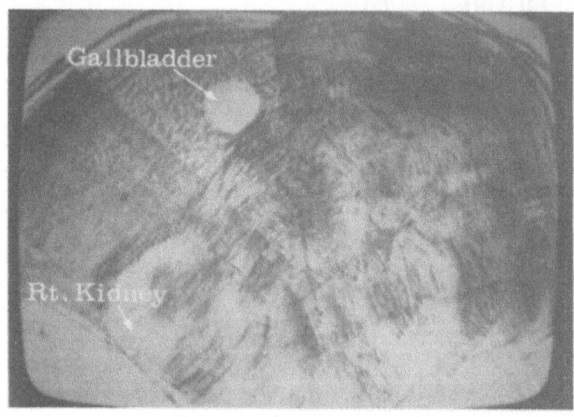

FIGURE 2.27
Supine transverse scan. The gallbladder becomes distended after an overnight fast. This echo-free structure may then be used as an anatomic reference point, and the contraction following a fatty meal better evaluated.

FIGURE 2.28 (a)
Supine transverse scan. Echo-free ovoid region at the undersurface of the liver. The gallbladder must be studied in two planes in order to document its characteristic shape and avoid confusion with other anechoic structures of similar size. Note the sharply outlined distal wall.

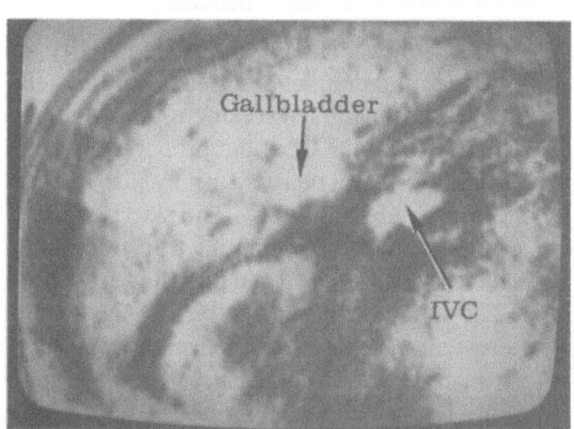

screen. After local anesthesia, the needle is advanced into the lesion to a predetermined depth. The contents of the suspected metastases are then aspirated and submitted for cytologic examination.

Sonography provides a sensitive and atraumatic method for localizing and diagnosing suspected metastatic foci. The percutaneous puncture technique permits simple histologic confirmation of suspected lesions.

THE GALLBLADDER

Current radiologic diagnosis of the biliary tract and gallbladder is very accurate, if these structures can be opacified by excreted contrast media. Ultrasonic visualization is unrelated to the functional status of this system and diseases of the gallbladder may be evaluated in the presence of a radiographically nonfunctioning gallbladder. This bears added importance since only 20 percent of gallstones are sufficiently radiopaque to be visualized on plain abdominal films.

Application of gray-scale systems and real-time scanners permits better evaluation of the dilated hepatobiliary system and offers a noninvasive alternative to percutaneous transhepatic cholangiography.

ANATOMY

The right and left hepatic ducts join at the porta hepatis to form the common hepatic duct, which becomes the common bile duct after giving off the cystic duct to the gallbladder. The common bile duct passes anterior to the inferior vena cava and through the superior aspect of the pancreatic head to enter the duodenum at the papilla of Vater.

The gallbladder is a distensible sac lying in a fossa on the inferior surface of the right hepatic lobe. The neck of the gallbladder and cystic duct are near the porta hepatis, while the fundus projects inferolaterally beyond the liver

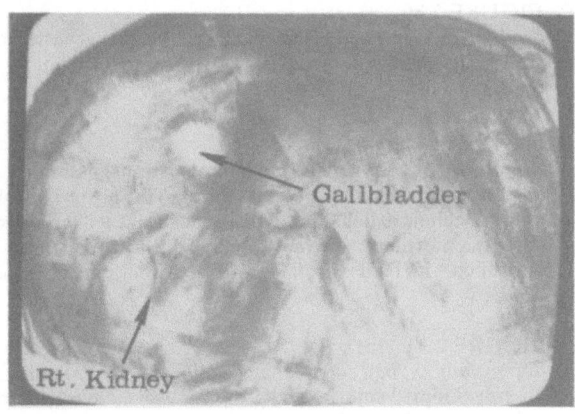

FIGURE 2-28 (b)

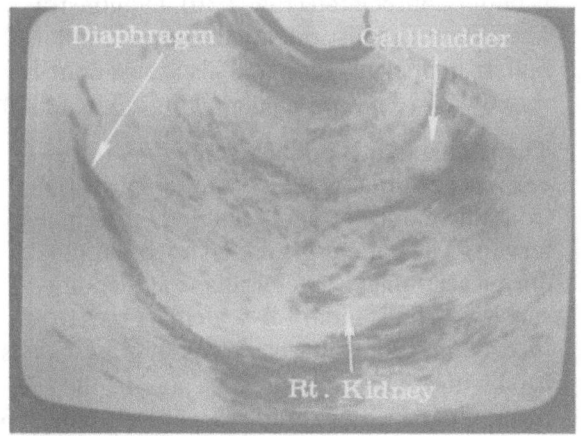

FIGURE 2-29 (a)

FIGURE 2-29 (b)

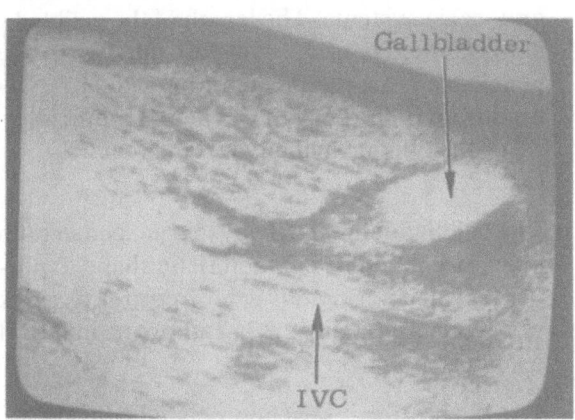

edge. The fundus may contact the anterior abdominal wall. Medially, it lies against the superior duodenum. Posteriorly, it is in relation to the transverse colon and upper pole of the right kidney. Laterally, the gallbladder lies in the concavity of the liver.

SONOANATOMY

The fluid-filled gallbladder appears echo free at low and medium sensitivities. It loses its anechoic pattern on B-scan if its anteroposterior diameter is less than 2.0 cm. The better resolution of gray-scale systems permits easier localization of the gallbladder in difficult cases and fluid-filled compartments greater than 1.5 cm wide (Fig. 2.27) can be imaged. The gallbladder is demonstrated along the inferior surface of the liver as an oval or round echo-free structure (Fig. 2.28a and b) and is roughly elliptical in its longitudinal axis (Fig. 2.29a and b).

In the filled gallbladder the posterior wall is sharply demarcated and can be delineated in one scan sweep. As it extends caudally, the gallbladder becomes more lateral and superficial. The nonfilled gallbladder is ill defined and difficult to localize.

SONOLAPAROTOMY

The patient is instructed to fast overnight to distend the gallbladder optimally (Fig. 2.27). The dilated gallbladder is more easily visual-

FIGURE 2.28 (b)
Supine transverse scan. The echo-free gallbladder usually appears under the liver surface. To study its true lie, multiple planes may be needed.

FIGURE 2.29 (a)
Supine longitudinal scan. The echo-free gallbladder may appear elliptical or wedge-shaped. It passes under the liver towards the anterior abdominal wall and is usually situated anterior to the right kidney.

FIGURE 2.29 (b)
Supine longitudinal scan. The gallbladder usually lies in an oblique position. The neck of the gallbladder is often situated over the inferior vena cava.

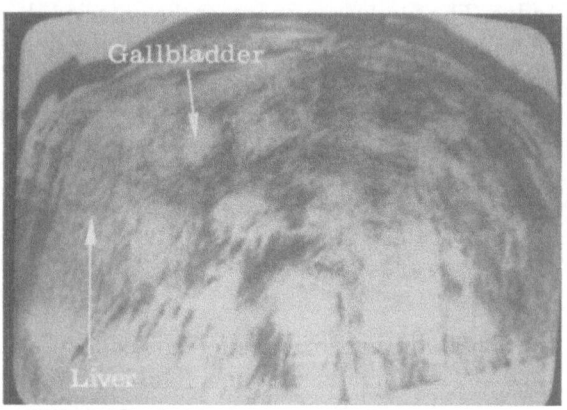

FIGURE 2-30

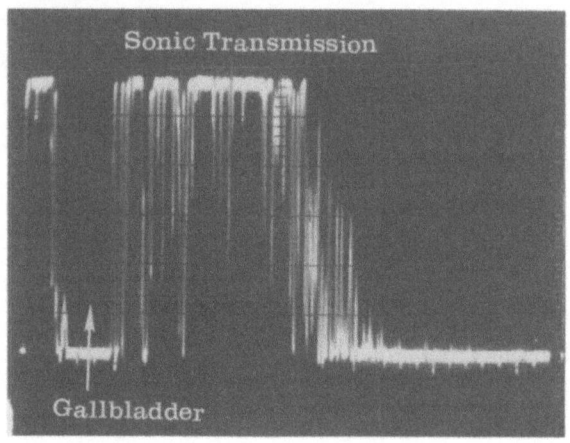

FIGURE 2-31 (a)

FIGURE 2-31 (b)

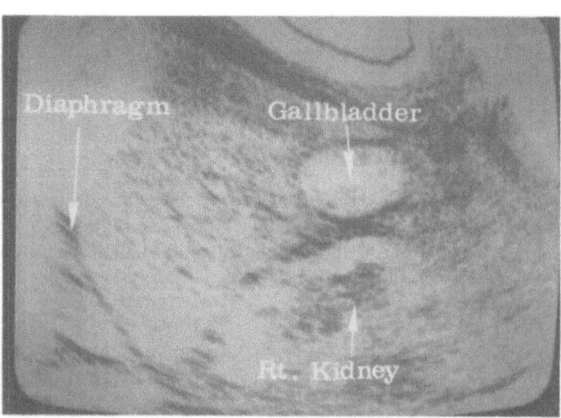

FIGURE 2.30
Supine transverse scan. The dilated gallbladder is easier to study. The gallbladder must be at least 1.5 cm in diameter to be imaged.

FIGURE 2.31 (a)
A-mode at high sensitivity. High through transmission demonstrated as multiple echoes distal to the posterior wall of the anechoic gallbladder. No change in size will be noted when the transducer is over the gallbladder. A duodenal bulb filled with fluid will change in size with normal contractions.

FIGURE 2.31 (b)
Supine longitudinal scan. Dilated gallbladder over kidney. Sharply outlined anterior and posterior walls. No response to fatty meal. Acute cholecystitis.

ized and contraction from a fatty meal stimulus is better appreciated (Fig. 2.30). Demonstration of contractility distinguishes the duodenal bulb from the gallbladder. This is best done by A-mode or real-time scanner (Fig. 2.31a and b).

The gallbladder is initially studied by transverse scans, followed by longitudinal sections from the midline towards the right in 1-cm intervals. The patient is told to stop breathing during scanning. Search is made at medium sensitivity on standard B-scan machines to detect round, echo-free structures. If gray scale is used with a linear method of scanning, the gallbladder can be more readily localized. When an echo-free region is identified in transverse scanning, oblique scans are made to outline the gallbladder along its maximum axis. The sensitivity setting is decreased at this point to prevent anterior-wall echo artifacts common to B-scanning equipment. No adjustments are made with gray-scale systems. The length of the gallbladder is marked over the skin with ink or a grease pencil and cross-section cuts are taken from the fundus up to the neck, if possible. In difficult cases the oblique maneuver is of great help (Fig. 2.32).

The gallbladder must always be imaged in both planes to obtain its characteristic shape to prevent misdiagnosing this echo-free area as a cyst of the pancreas (Fig. 2.33a and b) or a metastatic focus in the liver.

The biliary tree is best appreciated with gray-

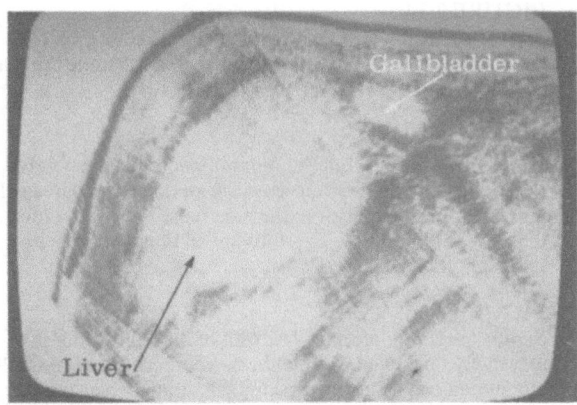

FIGURE 2-32

FIGURE 2.32
Supine oblique scan. The gallbladder was not imaged in the routine scanning planes. Partial outline of the gallbladder appears when the oblique scanning plane is used to localize this structure.

FIGURE 2.33   (a)
Supine longitudinal scan. Anechoic pancreatic pseudocyst simulating a normal elliptical gallbladder. This problem is solved when scanning in multiple planes to demonstrate the typical three-dimensional shape of the gallbladder.

FIGURE 2.33   (b)
Supine transverse scan. The round anechoic gallbladder, with a smooth distal wall, sits adjacent to a larger sonolucent region with an irregular distal border. Pancreatic pseudocyst.

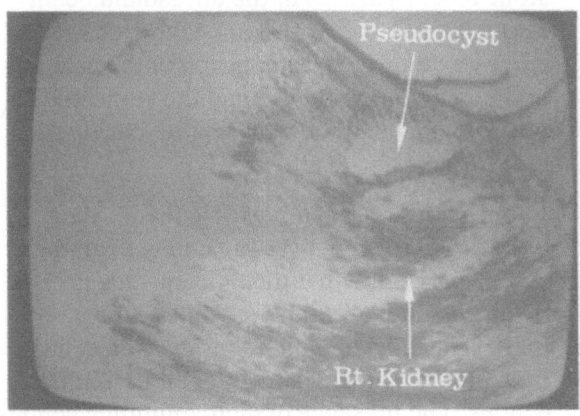

FIGURE 2-33 (a)

FIGURE 2-33 (b)

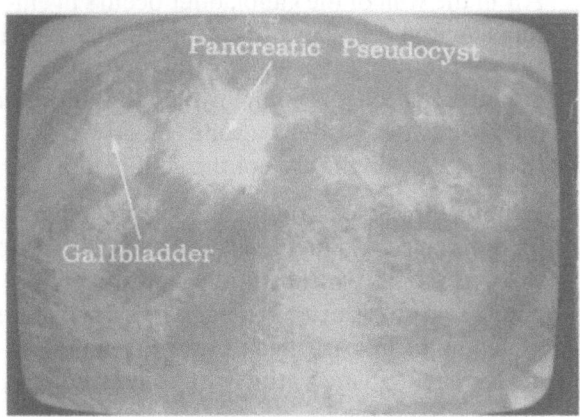

scale or real-time scanners. The ductal system must be dilated to 1.0 cm to be imaged clearly.

SONOPATHOLOGY

Congenitally, the gallbladder is only rarely absent. However, it may be on a mesenteric pedicle and located in areas other then the right upper quadrant. The entire abdomen must then be searched. Serosal and mucosal bands produce septations of the fundus. These sacculations may be confused with intraluminal disease, due to current resolution limitations of present ultrasonic equipment. The close proximity of the fundus to the fluid-filled duodenal bulb may produce a pseudoseptation or echogenic region (12). Repositioning may separate the duodenum, or rescanning might show peristaltic change in the duodenal bulb.

Primary acute cholecystitis is not associated with gallstones. An enlarged echo-free gallbladder is seen without internal echoes. There is no response to a fatty meal. Stones are present in chronic cholecystitis and vary from "gravel" to several centimeters in dimension. In the supine position, gallstones lie against the posterior wall and appear as echoes within the gallbladder. On B-scan, single or multiple echoes, close to the posterior wall, are noted. With gray-scale imaging, stones as small as 0.4 cm may be visualized as dark-gray masses of echoes adjacent to the distal wall (Fig. 2.34). With careful linear scan-

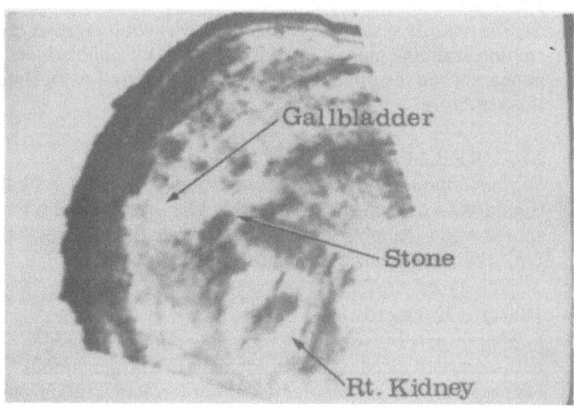

FIGURE 2-34

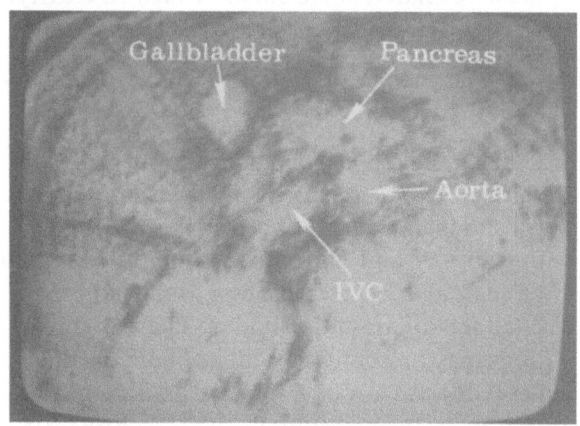

FIGURE 2-35

FIGURE 2-36

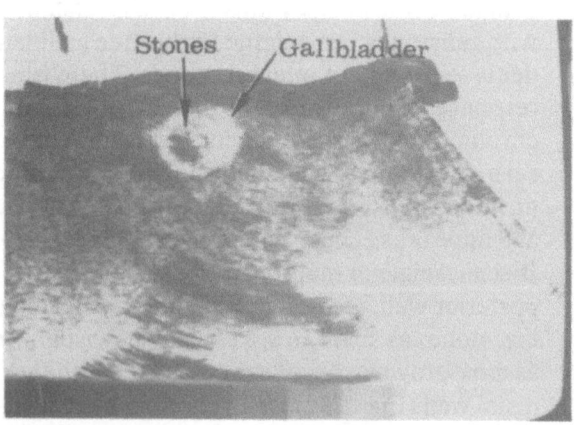

FIGURE 2.34
Supine transverse scan. The gallbladder is echo free. On the distal wall, high-amplitude echoes of a gallstone are noted. A sonic shadow occurs distal to the stone.

FIGURE 2.35
Supine transverse scan. Echo-poor pancreatic mass noted anterior to the inferior vena cava. A moderately dilated gallbladder appears anterior to the pancreas. The gallbladder did not contract following a fatty meal. Pancreatitis with reflex cholecystitis.

FIGURE 2.36
Supine longitudinal scan. The wall of the gallbladder is massively thickened. Within the remaining lumen are small stones and echogenic inspissated bile. Patient was not jaundiced. Carcinoma of the gallbladder. Head is toward the right.

ning, a sonic shadow may be produced as the stone blocks passage of the ultrasound beam (33). Distal to the stone is an echo-free space corresponding to the dimension of the calculus in the scanning plane. Behind the stone, the posterior gallbladder wall is either poorly seen or not visualized at all.

In one series the accuracy of gallstone detection was 89 percent by x-ray cholecystography and 72 percent with ultrasonic imaging (22). If the gallbladder is completely filled with stones, there is insufficient fluid to produce an echo-free interface in which to detect intraluminal echoes. The presence of high-amplitude echoes in the region of the gallbladder and the appearance of the sonic shadow (33) suggest a stone-filled lumen. In chronic cholecystitis, the gallbladder may be shrunken secondary to fibrosis and may contain too little fluid to be detected.

Air in the wall of the gallbladder occurs in emphysematous cholecystitis and air in the lumen is seen following certain surgical procedures. Air strongly reflects sound waves and this interface will either produce a sonic shadow or reflect artifacts in the area of the gallbladder.

In both chronic obstruction and acute inflammation the gallbladder is dilated and there is no response to fatty meal stimulus. Although the clinical setting is usually diagnostic, the pancreas should be investigated to rule out tumor mass or acute pancreatitis with reflex cholecystitis (Fig. 2.35).

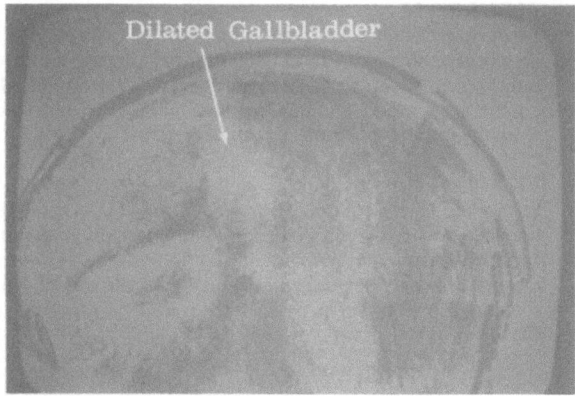

FIGURE 2-37 (a)

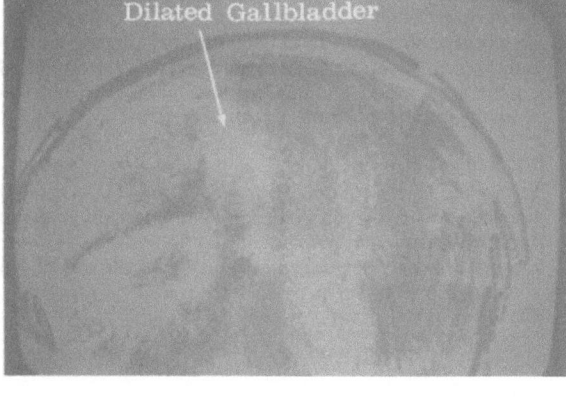

FIGURE 2-37 (b)

FIGURE 2-38

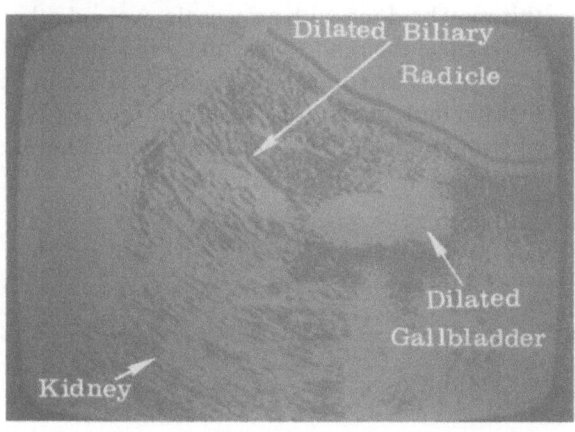

FIGURE 2.37 (a)
Supine transverse scan. The enlarged gallbladder is most commonly produced by common bile duct obstruction. The distended gallbladder will not respond to a fatty meal stimulus when there is distal obstruction.

FIGURE 2.37b (b)
Supine longitudinal scan. The enlarged gallbladder of the same patient. This distended gallbladder may simulate a cystic lesion from the liver or biliary ducts.

FIGURE 2.38
Supine longitudinal scan. The dilated common bile duct must be at least 1 cm to be imaged by gray scale. It may be distinguished from the portal vein by absence of pulsations, with the real-time scanner.

Carcinoma of the gallbladder is rare and generally associated with cholelithiasis or inspissated bile (Fig. 2.36). The diffusely infiltrating nature of this tumor usually prevents sufficient dilation of the gallbladder walls to be visualized as a separate fluid-filled structure. Papillomas are generally less than 1 cm in size and various hyperplastic changes of the mucosa are too small to image with the present system.

THE BILIARY TREE

SONOPATHOLOGY

Congenital weakness of the wall of the common bile duct and distal obstruction produce the choledochal cyst, which is a dilation of the extrahepatic biliary tract. This appears as an echo-free structure in the region of the porta hepatis, which does not respond to fatty meal stimulus. The clinical setting is characteristic.

Obstruction of the distal common bile duct is usually caused by impacted gallstones, carcinoma of the head of the pancreas, strictures of the common bile duct, lymphadenopathy, and secondary tumor deposits in the porta hepatis. Carcinoma of the common bile duct is rare.

Gradual obstruction causes proximal dilatation of the gallbladder (Fig. 2.37a and b), the common bile duct (Fig. 2.38), and intrahepatic biliary tree (Fig. 2.39). The enlarged common bile

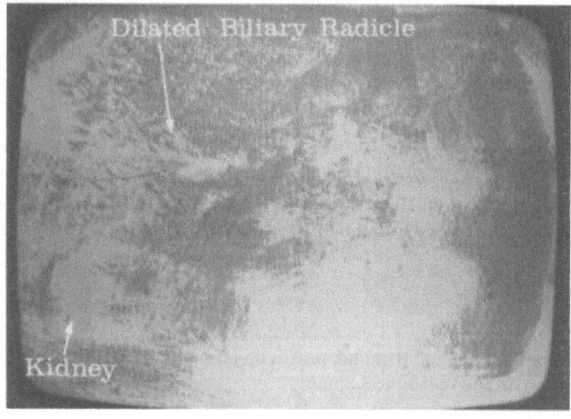

FIGURE 2-39

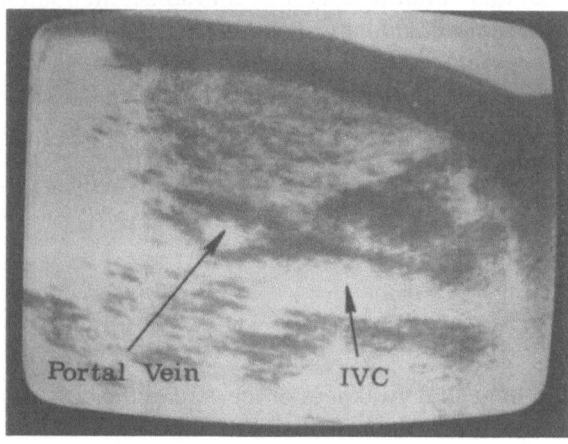

FIGURE 2-40

FIGURE 2.39
Supine transverse scan. Dilatation of the biliary system
may be detected in the liver bed as linear, tubular, echo-free
structures. Enlarged biliary radicles must be followed to the
confluence with the common hepatic duct for differentiation
from the intrahepatic portal venous system.

FIGURE 2.40
Supine longitudinal scan. The ovoid portal vein may be distinguished from an enlarged common bile duct by noting its
confluence from the splenic vein and the superior mesenteric vein. This may be performed with gray-scale or real-time
scanner. Note typical location of the portal vein anterior to
the inferior vena cava.

duct appears as a tubular echo-free structure on
longitudinal section, connecting with the dilated
branching echo-free major biliary radicles located cephalad (79).

The dilated common bile duct must be differentiated from the portal vein (Fig. 2.40). According to some investigators, the enlarged portal
vein is imaged as a comma-shaped, echo-free
structure with low-level intraluminal echoes
representing backscatter from red blood cells.
To support this diagnosis, the liver is examined
for increased echo density indicative or cirrhosis and the spleen studied for splenomegaly,
with medium level echoes characterizing
congestive splenic pathology. These findings
are best evaluated with gray scale (79).

We prefer to identify the portal vein by observing its formation from the splenic and superior
mesenteric venous tributaries. The splenic vein
posterior to the pancreas is first demonstrated
and then followed to the right upper quadrant to
its confluence with the portal vein. Although
this may be done with gray scale, we and others
(84) utilize the real-time scanner for speed and
accuracy. The superior mesenteric vein can be
located more accurately when the outflow is
obstructed and other conditions slow venous
return, such as portal vein thrombosis.

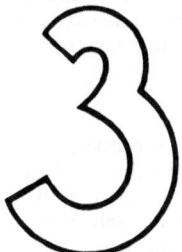

splenic sonography

GENERAL INTRODUCTION

The well-trained sonographer can image most of the spleen by ultrasound. Many pathologic conditions are manifested directly or indirectly as changes in splenic size or consistency. Thus, study of the spleen helps the examiner to evaluate various diseases.

The sonographer has the same responsibility as the pathologist slicing a surgical specimen. Extensive past experience with pathologic disorders of the spleen is extremely helpful in interpreting sonic sectional studies of the spleen. Ultrasonic examination of the spleen is especially important, since it is highly diagnostic of certain diseases and may save the patient from other diagnostic procedures with their greater morbidity and discomfort.

THE SPLEEN

ANATOMY

The spleen is located in the left upper quadrant of the abdomen under the left hemidiaphragm. The diaphragmatic

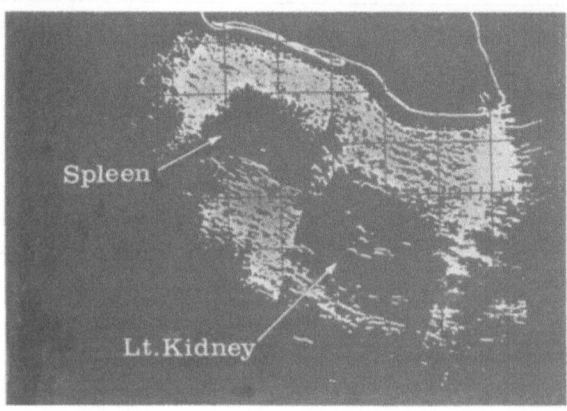

FIGURE 3-1 (a)

FIGURE 3.1 (a)
Prone longitudinal scan. B-mode at medium sensitivity. Echo-free spleen with high through transmission is compared with the slightly echogenic renal parenchyma situated caudally. The spleen fills-in with echoes only at very high sensitivity.

FIGURES 3.1 (b)
Prone longitudinal scan. High sensitivity study showing the renal parenchyma to fill in with echoes while the spleen remains sonolucent. Highest sensitivity settings must be used to fill-in the spleen. A-mode evaluation is useful in differentiating spleen from cystic mass.

FIGURE 3.2
A-mode at medium sensitivity. Echo-free zone denotes splenic parenchyma. Tall distal spike is the inner splenic wall. Note high through transmission. The spleen fills in with echoes at very high gain settings.

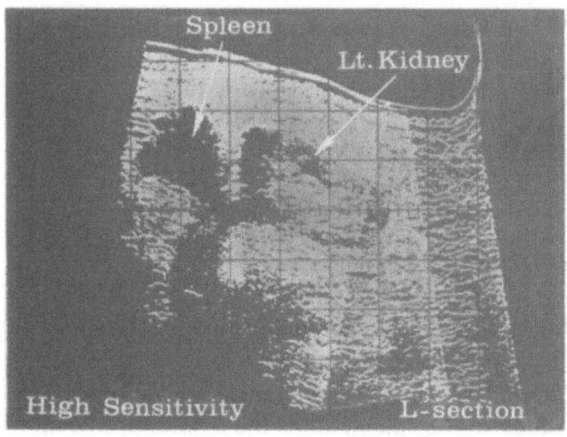

FIGURE 3-1 (b)

FIGURE 3-2

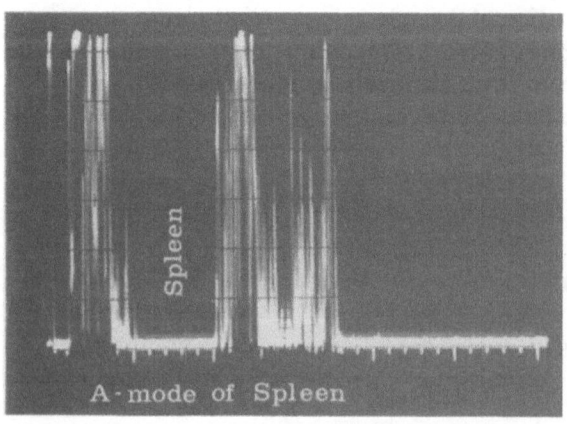

surface is smooth and convex. The visceral border is concave, with grooves facing the posterior stomach, lateral border of the left kidney, and tail of the pancreas. This roughly triangular-shaped organ has a centrally located hilus on the visceral surface, which contains the splenic vessels and lienorenal ligament. The anterior extension of the gland may be notched. The splenic vein crosses the posterior aspect of the pancreatic tail and body to join the inferior mesenteric vein and becomes the portal vein. The splenic artery is tortuous but generally lies anterior to the tail of the pancreas. The spleen is a distensible organ, and splenic volume varies with body activity and circulating blood volume.

SONOANATOMY

The normal spleen appears as a concave sonolucent structure in the left upper quadrant. The splenic pulp is homogeneous and the organ fills-in with echoes at very high sensitivity settings. It is much more sonolucent than the liver and slightly more sonolucent than the renal parenchyma (Fig. 3.1a and b). On the A-scope high-amplitude spikes mark the anterior and posterior borders (Fig. 3.2). Gray scale demonstrates the spleen as either anechoic or with light shades of gray, compared to the darker gray

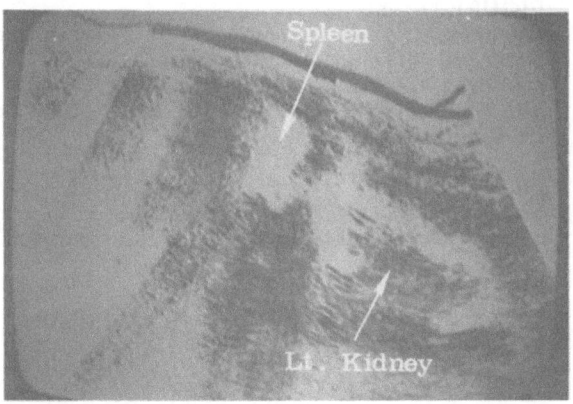

FIGURE 3-3

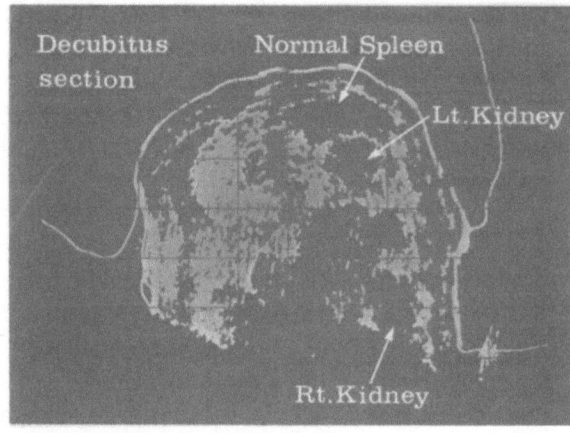

FIGURE 3-4

FIGURE 3-5

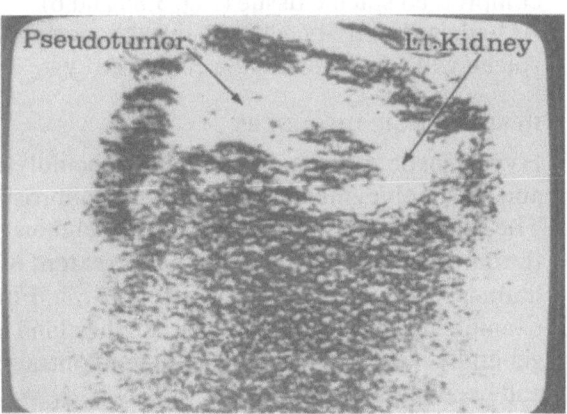

FIGURE 3.3
Prone longitudinal scan. The echo-poor parenchyma of the spleen is contrasted with the dark-gray echoes of the renal collecting system and the light-gray echoes from the renal cortex.

FIGURE 3.4
Left lateral decubitus scan. The spleen may be separated from the left kidney in this position. The spleen is scanned most easily from the transverse or oblique intercostal approach when the patient lies with the right side down.

FIGURE 3.5
Prone longitudinal scan. The pseudotumor of the kidney is easily produced by linear scanning techniques. Increasing the sensitivity may differentiate the parenchyma of the spleen from that of a cyst.

renal cortex (Fig. 3.3). The spleen covers the left kidney laterally and is located posteriorly and laterally in relation to the stomach. The splenic vein courses along the pancreas posteriorly and appears as a linear echo-free structure on gray-scale images. This vein is pulsatile with the real-time scanner.

SONOLAPAROTOMY

The position of the patient for scanning depends upon the size of the spleen. Large spleens can always be demonstrated in the supine position; small spleens are very difficult to study properly but, with maximum effort, this organ may be imaged in the left lateral decubitus (Fig. 3.4) or prone position. In the decubitus position the transducer is moved transversely or oblique intercostally to image the spleen optimally. The pseudotumor of the kidney is easily produced by linear scanning over the upper pole of the left kidney (Fig. 3.5). The spleen can be differentiated from a cyst by increasing sensitivity. To adequately demarcate the spleen from the left upper pole a useful, prone, scanning technique is to sector scan when approaching the splenorenal interface (Fig. 3.6a and b). Occasionally a distended stomach permits better visualization of the spleen. During scanning, the patient is instructed to stop breathing.

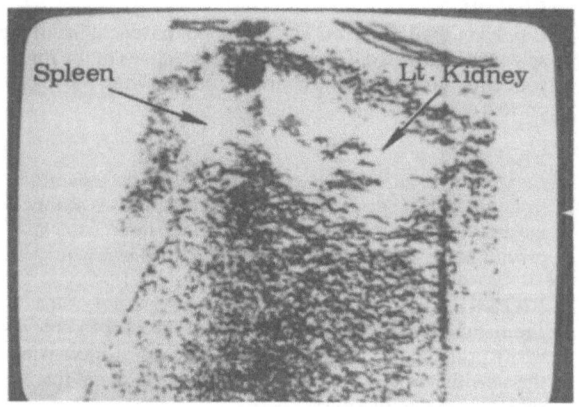

FIGURE 3-6 (a)

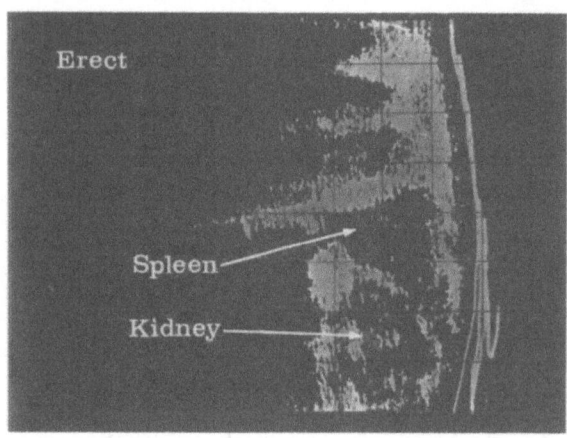

FIGURE 3-6 (b)

FIGURE 3-7

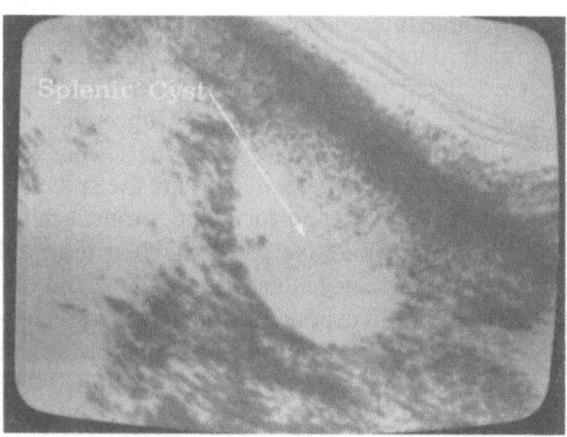

FIGURE 3.6 (a)
Prone longitudinal scan. The spleen may be separated from the upper pole of the left kidney by decubitus positions. A useful maneuver to demarcate the spleen from the upper pole of the kidney is sector scanning when approaching the splenorenal interface.

FIGURE 3.6 (b)
Erect longitudinal scan. This position may be used to separate the spleen from the kidney. Sector scanning is useful.

FIGURE 3.7
Prone longitudinal scan. Echo-free zone represents acquired splenic cyst. Smooth distal wall.

SONOPATHOLOGY

ANOMALIES

Congenital variations of the spleen include asplenia, splenic separations, accessory spleens, and polysplenia with multiple small spleens. Rather large spleens have been incidentally noted as a normal variation in both adults and children.

CYSTS

True cysts of the spleen are rare and may be due to parasites (Echinococcus) or teratoma. False cysts are more common and usually occur in the young adult. They may be serous or hemorrhagic and are believed to represent organizing hematomas (46,69). The cyst has a sharp posterior border and high through transmission (Fig. 3.7). If the cyst is hemorrhagic or septate, internal echoes may be demonstrated. An attempt is made to visualize the remaining compressed splenic tissue (Fig. 3.8a and b). At higher sensitivity settings, the echongenic spleen will contrast with the echo-free cyst.

HEMATOLOGIC DISORDERS

Hyperplastic splenomegaly occurs in hemolytic anemias, polycythemia vera, and myelofibrosis. The size and internal echo pattern depend on the chronicity of the disorder and the extent of fibrosis or calcification of the parenchyma. For example, in early sickle cell disease the gland is generally large and anechoic but later contracts and becomes echogenic.

Primary malignant tumors of the spleen are in

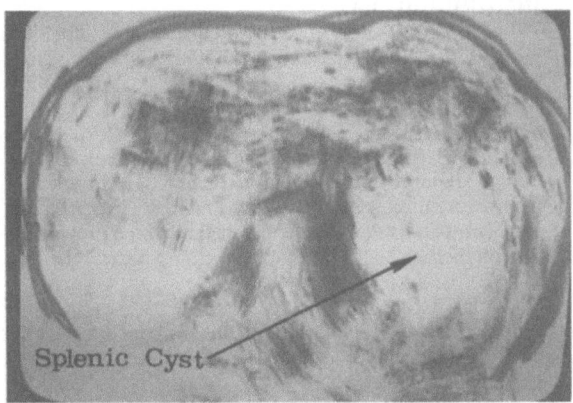

FIGURE 3-8 (a)

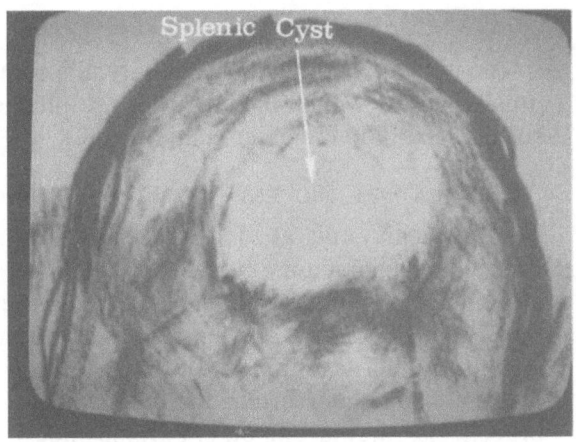

FIGURE 3-8 (b)

FIGURE 3-9

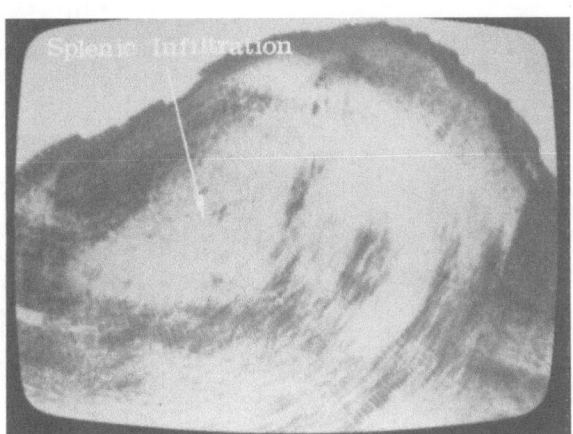

FIGURE 3.8 (a)
Supine transverse scan. Large echo-free cyst occupies left upper quadrant. Distal wall sharply outlined.

FIGURE 3.8 (b)
Left decubitus scan. The echo-free splenic cyst is well demonstrated. This type of cyst may simulate the cyst of the upper pole of left kidney. Several views are needed for verification.

FIGURE 3.9
Left lateral decubitus scan. The enlarged spleen markedly attenuates the sound beam. As a result the distal border is poorly outlined. The spleen is echo-poor. This appearance may be seen in lymphomatous infiltration of the spleen.

the lymphoma family. The spleen may contain discrete foci of tumor, with or without necrosis. In advanced disease complete replacement of the organ may occur. Multiple foci of tumor may appear echogenic. The diffusely infiltrated spleen is homogeneous and generally anechoic unless areas of necrosis exist. Most of these spleens highly attenuate the ultrasound beam so that the posterior border is poorly demonstrated (Fig. 3.9). Differentiation of this echo-free tumor from a cyst depends upon the through transmission pattern (31).

In leukemia cellular infiltration is diffuse. Small spleens are generally noted in acute leukemia, while larger spleens occur in chronic leukemia. Infarction and fibrosis are more common in chronic myelogenous leukemia than in chronic lymphatic leukemia. These spleens tend to have anechoic or low-level echo-producing parenchyma. However, we have observed echogenic spleens in chronic myelogenous leukemia (Fig. 3.10a and b).

TRAUMA

The enlarged spleen is more easily traumatized. The lacerated spleen will usually maintain its size and shape as blood spills intraperitoneally. If the capsule is intact, a splenic hematoma will result, enlarging and distorting the splenic outline (Fig. 3.11a and b). Following trauma, inspection is made for intraperitioneal blood. The spleen is examined for breaks in the continuity of the cortical outline or areas of hemorrhage that appear separated from the normal tissue by a band of echoes corresponding to the blood-

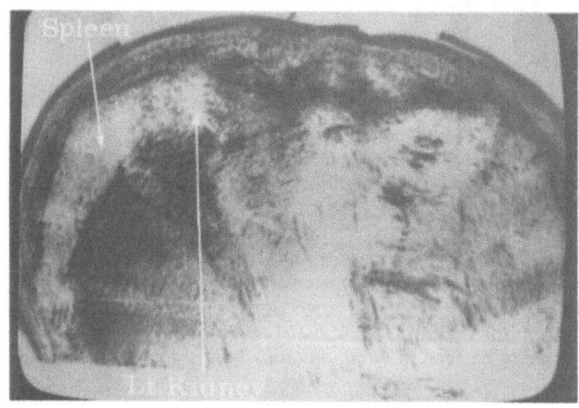

FIGURE 3-10 (a)

FIGURE 3.10 (a)
Prone transverse scan. The enlarged spleen is slightly echogenic. Little sound attenuation is noted. Chronic myelogenous leukemia.

FIGURE 3.10 (b)
Left lateral decubitus scan. The spleen is more echogenic than the renal cortex. This pattern is noted in chronic inflammatory diseases of the spleen and in the irradiated organ. This patient, with leukemia, had received previous radiation therapy.

FIGURE 3.10 (c)
Supine transverse scan. The spleen is enlarged, echo poor and transonic. The spleen crosses the midline of the body. Chronic leukemia.

FIGURE 3.11 (a)
Supine transverse scan. Splenic hematoma without break in the capsule will diffusely enlarge the organ. Spontaneous splenic hematoma in patient with Gaucher's disease.

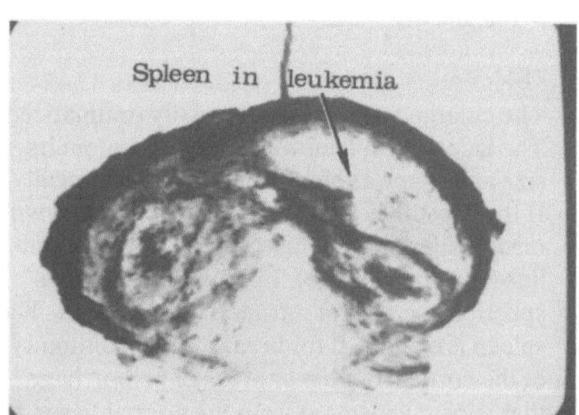

FIGURE 3-10 (b)

spleen interface. At higher sensitivity, the compressed spleen will fill-in with echoes, while the subcapsular blood remains echo free (37).

INFLAMMATORY PROCESS

The spleen may enlarge in the presence of extrasplenic inflammatory disease or may be the site of septic infarcts resulting in abscess formation. Splenic abscesses may appear as irregular sonolucent foci as the spleen becomes sonopaque at higher gain settings. Tuberculosis, brucellosis, sarcoid, and other chronic infections tend to produce echogenic spleens (77).

FIGURE 3-10 (c)

FIGURE 3-11 (a)

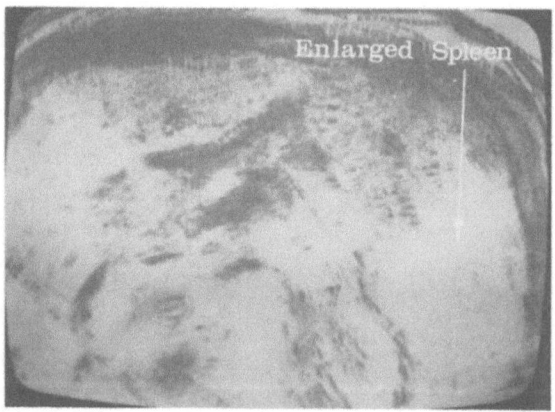

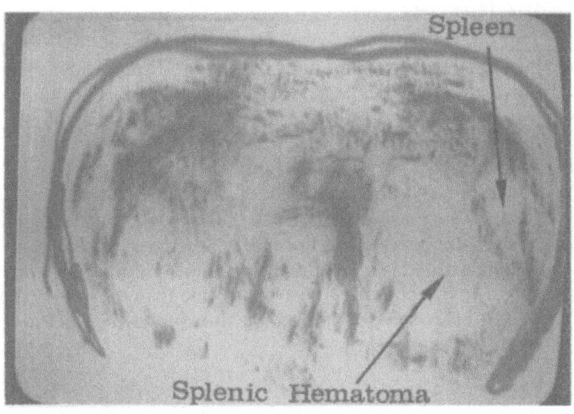

FIGURE 3-11 (b)

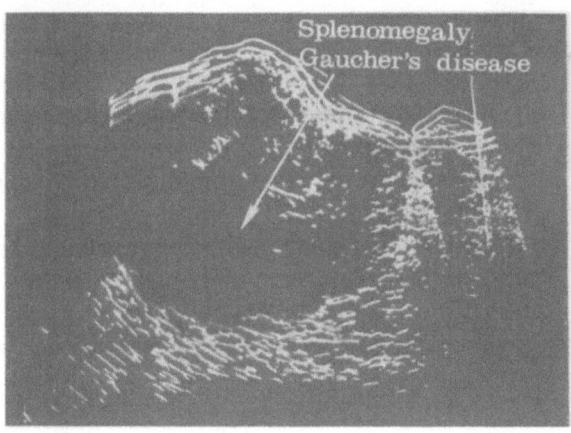

FIGURE 3-12 (a)

FIGURE 3-12 (b)

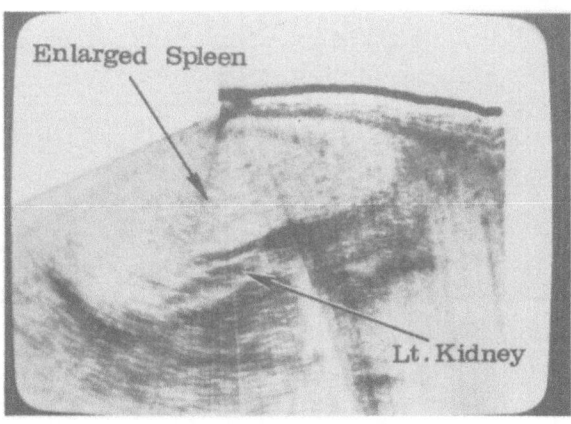

FIGURE 3.11 (b)
Supine transverse scan. The spleen is displaced laterally and anteriorly by a massive hematoma. Hematoma is echo free.

FIGURE 3.12 (a)
Supine longitudinal scan. Enlarged spleen with scattered regions of thick, high-amplitude echoes. These correspond to multiple areas of necrosis and fibrosis occurring in the infiltrated spleen of Gaucher's disease.

FIGURE 3.12 (b)
Supine longitudinal scan. The massively enlarged spleen with diffuse echogenic pattern. The kidney is compressed. Gaucher's disease.

INFILTRATIVE DISORDERS

In benign infiltrative disorders that cause deposition of metabolic products within the cells, such as Gaucher's disease, the enlarged spleen has an echo pattern consistent with the degree of internal necrosis and fibrosis. Our case material showed moderately echogenic parenchyma (Fig. 3.12a and b).

CONGESTION

Passive congestion of the spleen is common in chronic congestive heart failure, cirrhosis of the liver, and portal vein or splenic vein thrombosis or stenosis. The size of the spleen is generally moderate to large and the presence of medium-level internal echoes probably corresponds to the thickened trabeculae noted pathologically (76) (Fig. 3.13). When passive congestion is suspected, the echo pattern of the liver should be studied for cirrhotic changes and the presence of ascitic fluid investigated.

VOLUME DETERMINATION

In general, medical disease of the spleen diffusely enlarges the organ (46), while space-occupying lesions distort the splenic outline and compress normal parenchyma.

The spleen may be enormously enlarged and yet not project below the left costal margin (67). Splenic volume can be determined by analyzing the scans with a pencil-following device linked to a computer system (67). Massive splenomeg-

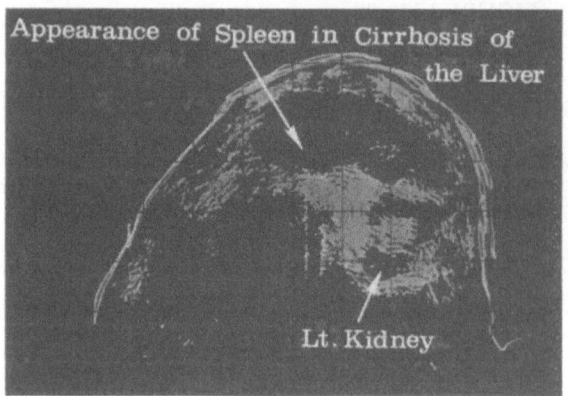

FIGURE 3-13 (a)

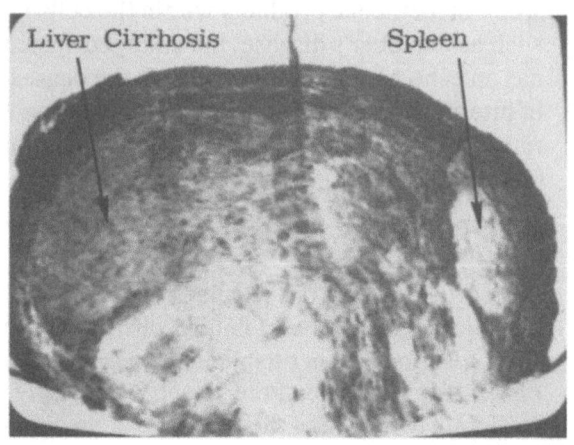

FIGURE 3-13 (b)

FIGURE 3-14

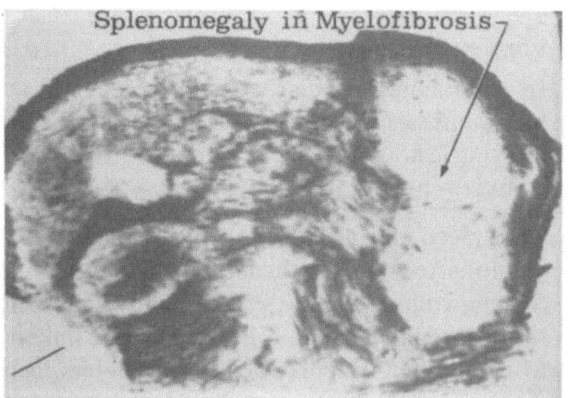

FIGURE 3.13   (a)
Left lateral decubitus scan. The spleen is moderately enlarged. Note the appearance of medium-level echoes. These correspond to pathologically thickened trabeculae characteristically observed in chronic passive congestion of the spleen. Cirrhosis of the liver.

FIGURE 3.13   (b)
Supine transverse scan. The liver is enlarged and echogenic to a greater degree than normal. A portion of the enlarged spleen is noted in a position more anterior than usual. The splenic parenchyma is more echogenic than the kidney due to chronic passive venous congestion in cirrhosis of the liver.

FIGURE 3.14
Supine transverse scan. The spleen is massively enlarged. This organ is transonic and a high through transmission pattern is demonstrated. A few scattered low-level echoes indicate areas of internal inhomogeneity. Myelofibrosis with splenomegaly.

aly occurs in chronic leukemia, portal hypertension, Gaucher's disease, Hodgkin's disease, myelofibrosis (Fig. 3.14), lymphosarcoma, and some chronic hemolytic anemias. Accurate determination of splenic volume is useful in the diagnosis and management of hematologic disorders.

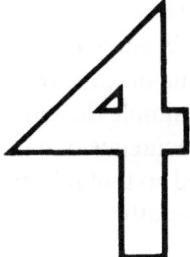

pancreatic sonography

GENERAL INTRODUCTION

Pancreatic lesions remain a difficult diagnostic problem. This is particularly true of chronic pancreatitis and tumors of the pancreas. Pancreatic pseudocysts·can be diagnosed indirectly only after they have exceeded a certain size and begin to displace air-filled structures in x-ray films of the abdomen or barium-filled bowel. Also, pseudocysts of the pancreas are frequently found in uncommon locations.

Radiologically, carcinoma of the head of the pancreas is frequently diagnosed when it is at an incurable stage. Tumors of the body and tail of the pancreas are difficult to detect clinically or radiographically. Angiography increases diagnostic accuracy, but superselective pancreatic arteriography entails significant risk to the patient and it may be difficult to differentiate inflammatory disease from malignant lesions. Isotope imaging of the pancreas is a helpful but not highly accurate diagnostic adjunct.

Pancreatic sonography is not only noninvasive but it has been used successfully to diagnose pancreatic pathology when all other studies failed. Serial examinations can be performed without risk or discomfort to the patient and are useful in documenting the size of the pancreas in acute pancreatitis and changes in its volume in exacerbations of chronic pancreatitis. A simple diagnostic test is essential, because the incidence of pancreatic carcinoma has increased so that it is now the fourth leading cause of death from cancer.

THE PANCREAS

ANATOMY

The pancreas lies obliquely in the anterior compartment of the retroperitoneum and is divided into a head, neck, body, and tail. It is usually several centimeters thick and approximately 14 cm in length in the adult.

The head of the pancreas sits in the curve of the duodenum. Dorsally situated, are the inferior vena cava, right renal vessels, and the left renal vein as it enters the inferior vena cava. A caudal projection of the head is the uncinate process, which the superior mesenteric vessels cross to reach the root of the mesentery. The common bile duct enters the duodenum by passing through the posterior substance of the pancreatic head.

The neck is an isthmus connecting the head of the pancreas to the body. The body is an inverted wedge-shaped structure, thin above and thick below. The anterior surface is covered by the stomach, whereas the posterior surface lies adjacent to the aorta, and (medial to lateral) the origin of the superior mesenteric artery, splenic vein, and left kidney.

The tail is the narrow segment extending towards the splenic hilum, often running in the base of the lienorenal ligament. Posteriorly, is the left kidney and splenic vein. The splenic artery courses superiorly; distally it turns anteriorly and runs ventral to the tail. (Fig. 4.1).

The pancreatic duct, which extends through the substance of the gland, is formed from the smaller ducts of the lobules. It enters the

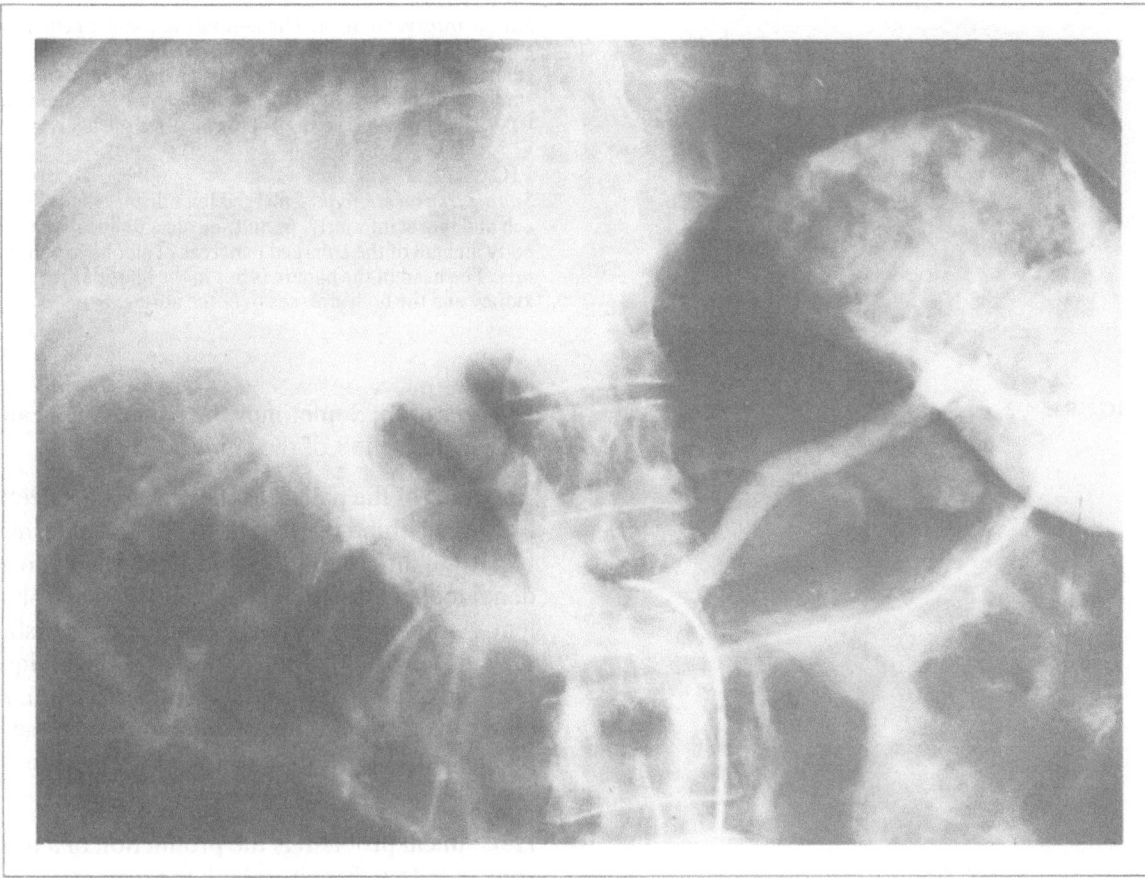

FIGURE 4.1
Venous phase of celiac arteriogram. The blush of the pancreas seen through the air-distended stomach permits good imaging. Note the size and shape of the pancreas. The junction of the splenic vein and portal vein occurs dorsal to the neck of the pancreas (courtesy of JJ Smulewicz M.D. and M Tafreshi M.D., Queens Hospital Center, Jamaica, N.Y.)

duodenum in proximity to the common bile duct.

SONOANATOMY

The pancreas has numerous blood vessels, ducts, and a lobular architecture. The many interfaces in this organ produce internal echoes at medium sensitivity. Sonographically, it is usually ill-defined due to the normal irregularity of the gland and the absence of a well-defined pancreatic capsule. The normal pancreas is more echogenic than the liver, spleen, or kidney. It has a "pebbly" gray echo pattern on gray-scale systems (Fig. 4.2). The location and shape of the pancreas vary considerably. It is positioned rather anteriorly and may assume a sigmoid, L-shaped, V-shaped, or horseshoe

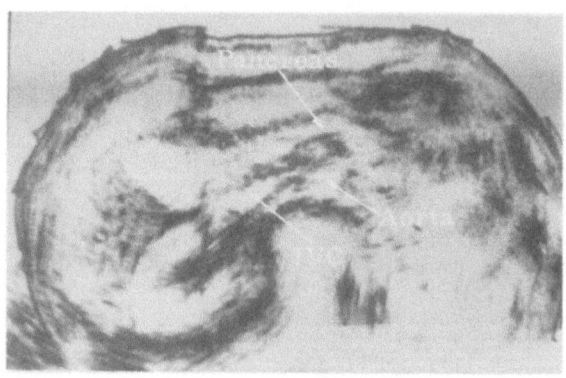

FIGURE 4-2

FIGURE 4.2
Supine transverse scan. The normal pancreas is generally situated beneath the inferior surface of the liver. The echogenic "cobblestone" appearance of the pancreatic substance is noted above the aorta and superior mesenteric artery. The pancreas is more echogenic than the liver.

FIGURE 4.3   (a)
Supine transverse scan. Enlarged liver displaces the stomach and bowel inferiorly, permitting clear delineation of the body and tail of the enlarged pancreas of alcoholic pancreatitis. The head of the pancreas lies in the hilus of the right kidney and the body crosses over the aorta.

configuration. Sometimes the pancreatic head may lie to the left of the spine.

The head of the pancreas may produce an echo-free area behind the liver (16). This is extremely hard to differentiate from a fluid-filled duodenal loop, and A-mode may clarify the problem. A significant obstacle in obtaining satisfactory visualization of the pancreas is the oblique position of the organ in the retroperitoneum. In either the standard longitudinal or transverse planes only a portion of the gland can be imaged.

A technical problem is the production of a transonic window through which the pancreas can be visualized, since the lower ribs, sternum, vertebrae, and air-containing structures (stomach, colon, lung) produce impediments to sonic transmission in all scanning positions. An attempt must be made to produce a suitable scanning window for optimal delineation of the pancreas.

There is a difference of opinion regarding visualization of the normal pancreas. Some authors believe that the normal pancreas is (43) essentially invisible with B-scanning systems, but any condition that causes edema of the pancreas or a space-occupying lesion permits visualization. Another group feels that the normal pancreas can be seen at low-gain settings, with a custom designed unit (37). In our experience the normal pancreas can be imaged occasionally with conventional B-scanners and frequently detected with gray-scale equipment. The normal pancreas is often better appreciated in the presence of hepatomegaly or other upper ab-

FIGURE 4-3 (a)

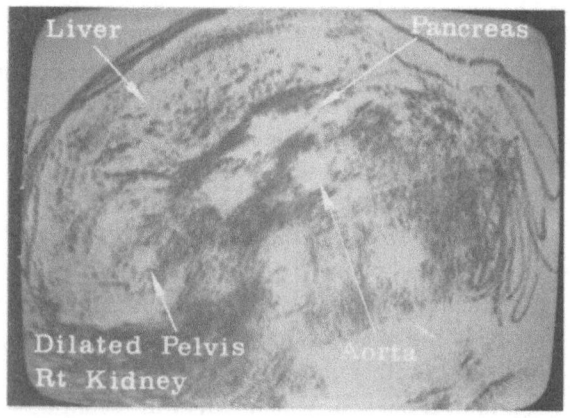

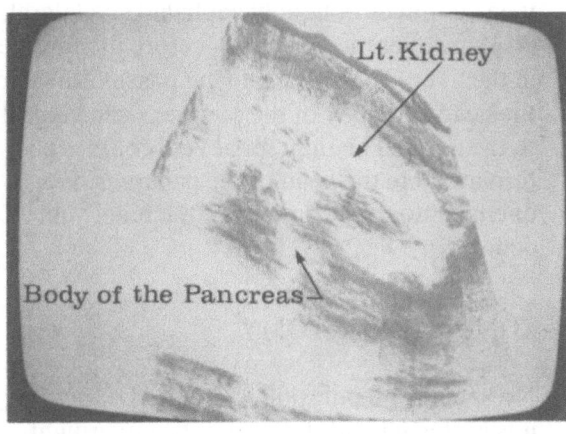

FIGURE 4-3 (b)

FIGURE 4.3   (b)
Prone longitudinal scan. The body and tail of the pancreas cross anterior to the left kidney and the gland appears as a small ovoid structure as scan is carried over the long axis of the kidney.

FIGURE 4.4
Supine transverse scan. The anechoic splenic vein is anterior to the aorta and inferior vena cava. This may be mistaken for the inflamed pancreas. The vein is distinguished from the gland by characteristic pulsations noted with the real-time scanner.

dominal mass that displaces the bowel inferiorly (Fig. 4.3a and b).

The resolution of real-time scanners and gray-scale units allows better definition of peripancreatic vasculature. Characteristic pulsations of vessels, with the real-time scanner, distinguish arteries from veins. The Valsalva maneuver will dilate venous structures imaged by the gray-scale system.

The aorta lies dorsal to the body of the pancreas. The superior mesenteric artery arises anteriorly from the aorta and passes behind the neck of the pancreas. It then turns anterior to the uncinate process of the pancreas and finally runs parallel with the abdominal aorta. The superior mesenteric artery, on cross-section appears, as a small echo-free lumen anterior to the aorta; in longitudinal scan, it looks like an echo-free tube above the aorta.

The superior mesenteric vein generally lies anterior and to the right of the superior mesenteric artery. This vein becomes larger near its junction with the splenic vein, to form the portal vein. At the level of the origin of the superior mesenteric artery, the superior mesenteric vein is several times the diameter of the artery and is situated dorsal to the pancreatic body. The splenic vein lies along the posterosuperior margin of the body and tail of the pancreas. The venous structures are echo free at standard gray-scale settings. The linear anechoic splenic vein, which crosses the aorta transversely, is often mistaken for the pancreas by the inexperienced sonographer (Fig. 4.4). The junction of the splenic and superior mesenteric veins lies behind the neck of the pancreas. The portal

FIGURE 4-4

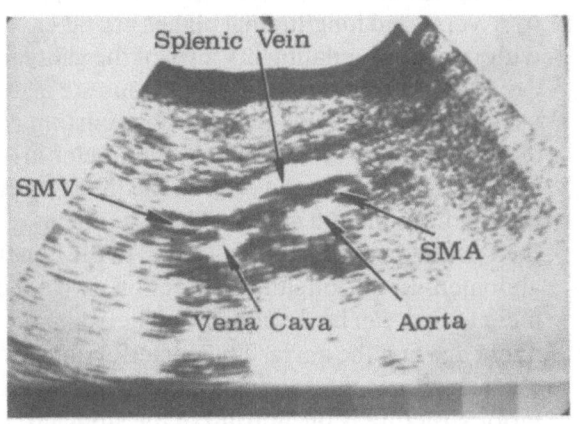

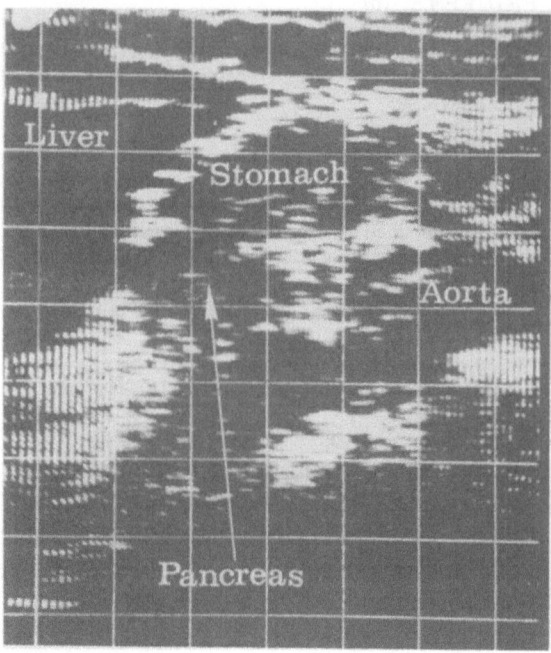

FIGURE 4.5 (a)
Supine longitudinal scan. The stomach is moderately distended with gasless water. The pancreas appears as an echo-free zone between the stomach and the aorta. The walls of the enlarged pancreas are seen due to acute pancreatitis.

FIGURE 4.5 (b)
Supine longitudinal scan. The stomach is distended with fluid and internal echoes represent retained food. The filled stomach serves as a scanning window to better image the pancreas. The enlarged head of the pancreas is echo-free due to pancreatitis.

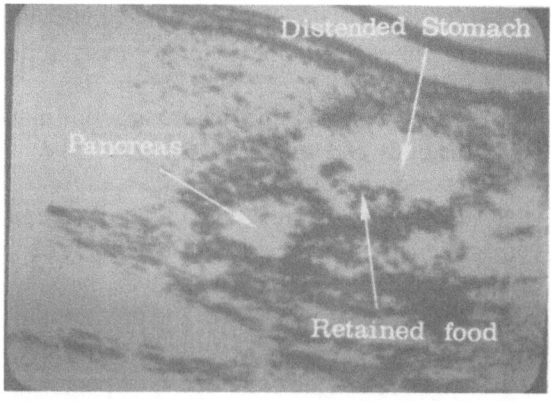

vein continues obliquely cephalad and lateral, crossing over the vena cava before it bifurcates in the liver. The left renal vein passes dorsal to the head and body of the pancreas and ventral to the aorta. The right renal vein courses posterolateral to the head of the pancreas. Frequent anatomic variations of the renal vein occur.

SONOLAPAROTOMY

No specific preparation is required. However, it is preferred that the patient fast overnight, since it is often necessary to pass a nasogastric tube to evacuate excess air or dilate the stomach with fluid during the scanning procedure before the body and tail of the pancreas can be seen (Fig. 4.5a and b). Fasting dilates the gallbladder, adding a useful anatomic reference point (Fig. 4.6). Radiographic contrast in the gastrointestinal tract may interfere with the study. Water-soluble contrast may produce echoes in the filled viscus, and barium completely blocks sound transmission in the gastrointestinal tract (50). Pancreatic disorders are better imaged in a well-hydrated patient (51). Excessive bowel gas creates a highly reflecting barrier to sound waves, and scanning must be postponed if other techniques to produce a sonic window fail. The use of Simethicone over a two-day period has been suggested as an effective method of reducing bowel gas (62).

The examination should be performed in the supine, prone, and decubitus positions and with varying sensitivities. Different sections in the transverse and longitudinal planes are taken with varying angulations. Views of the gallbladder and spleen in different projections are also useful. In scanning the pancreas our custom is to make transverse cuts at half-centimeter intervals along the plane between the hilum of the right kidney and the spleen. The scanning is then performed longitudinally across the upper abdomen. In the longitudinal section, two sonolucent areas can be demonstrated between the liver edge and the aorta. The posterior and cephalic region is the pancreas and the inferoanterior structure is the antrum of the stomach.

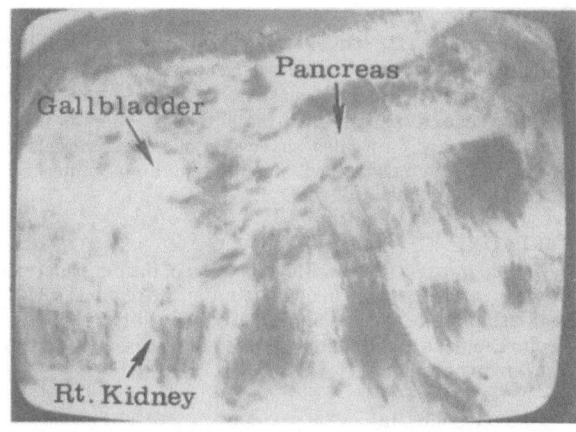

FIGURE 4.6
Supine transverse scan. The dilated gallbladder in the fasting patient adds a useful anatomic reference point for better evaluation of the pancreas. Enlarged pancreas from pancreatitis.

The transducer may be angled 10° to 20° caudal or cephalad, in the transverse or oblique sections, to maximize the amount of pancreatic tissue imaged. Tilting in the subcostal and intercostal scanning planes is often helpful. It is said that an oblique scan through the long axis of the pancreas may be obtained by placing the transducer parallel to the right costal margin, with a cephalic tilt of 20° to 30° (82). However, our experience reveals that multiple oblique sections, with varying angulations from the right hilum toward the spleen, are necessary to image the entire pancreas. After the pancreas has been localized, it is diagnostically helpful to study the gallbladder (43).

After maximum information is obtained from the supine position, the patient is turned to the prone position. Transverse and longitudinal sections are taken, focusing attention on the left flank, in the vicinity of the spleen, to image the tail of the pancreas.

If gray-scale or real-time scanners are not available, the following criteria for an adequate supine pancreatic B-scan (16) on cross-section scanning are necessary:

1. The posterior surface of the liver should be well demarcated.
2. The anterior surface of the spine is visualized.
3. The inferior vena cava and aorta are seen.
4. The stomach should not impede sonic transmission to the left paraspinal area.

On longitudinal scanning through transmission must be demonstrated by visualizing the angle between the inferior surface of the liver and the anterior surface of aorta or spine.

The pancreas may be localized more accurately by mapping the regional vascular anatomy. This is best accomplished with the real-time scanner, however, gray-scale machines offer sufficient resolution to detail venous landmarks. The origin of the superior mesenteric artery usually designates the cephalic border of the neck of the pancreas. Venous structures are best visualized in a cross-section study, starting

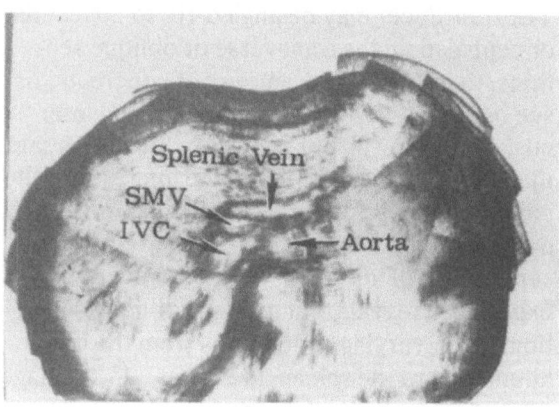

FIGURE 4-7 (a)

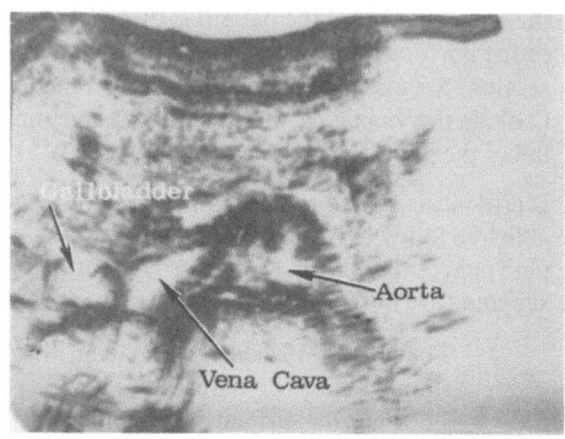

FIGURE 4-7 (b)

FIGURE 4-8 (a)

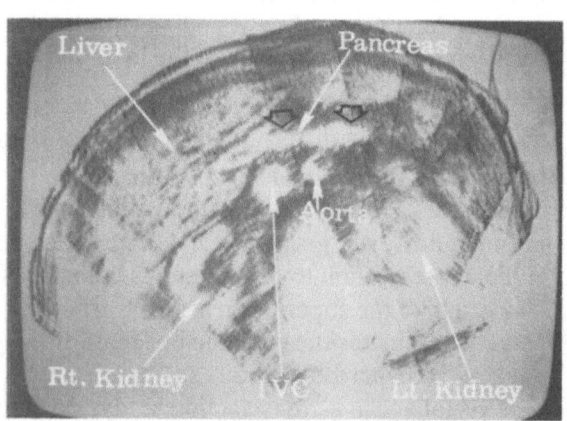

FIGURE 4.7 (a)
Supine transverse scan. Peripancreatic vasculature. Immediately anterior to the spine are the aorta and inferior vena cava. The ovoid superior mesenteric vein lies above the inferior vena cava and is much larger than the superior mesenteric artery. Crossing transversely over these vessels is the splenic vein, which will join the superior mesenteric vein to form the portal vein.

FIGURE 4.7 (b)
Supine transverse scan. Magnification of the peripancreatic region may be of help in demonstrating the regional relationships of the vessels to the surrounding organs. The anechoic lumens of the gallbladder, inferior vena cava, and aorta are in one plane.

FIGURE 4.8 (a)
Supine transverse scan. The acutely inflamed pancreas appears as a sonolucent band above the aorta and inferior vena cava. The edema of acute inflammation produces high through transmission and the margins of the gland are distinctly outlined. The distal wall is well seen.

from the xiphoid process and scanning caudally. The anechoic portal vein is sliced obliquely and appears to be ovoid in shape. As it is sectioned inferiorly, it moves medially and then receives the tubular splenic vein. This junction of the splenic vein with the superior mesenteric vein has a fixed relationship to the neck of the pancreas (70) (Fig. 4.7a and b).

Vascular anatomy is localized at low-gain settings with both gray-scale and real-time scanners. After the region of the pancreas is determined, the gain is increased to fill-in the parenchyma of the gland with medium-level echoes.

We have noted that the inferior vena cava cannot be well shown in transverse sections if the volume of the pancreas has increased; and there are also times the aorta cannot be visualized. Verification of the aorta may be made by M-mode, or real-time scanner.

SONOPATHOLOGY

PANCREATITIS

Sonography is extremely helpful in the acute stage of pancreatitis when the gland is edematous and usually well visualized (37). The best

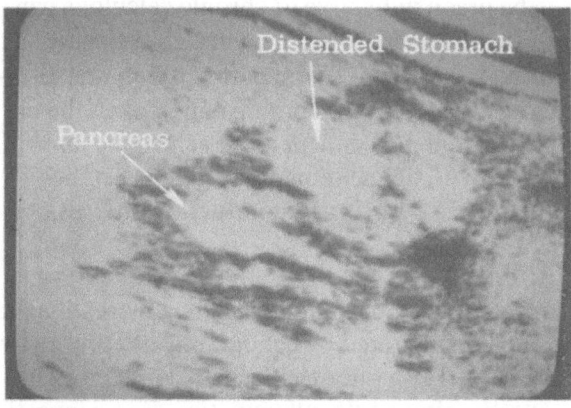

FIGURE 4-8 (b)

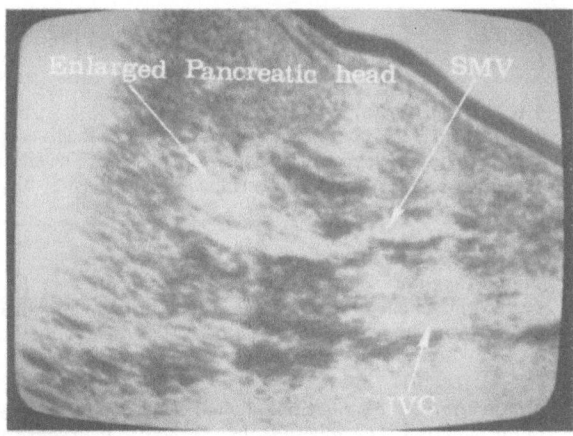

FIGURE 4-9 (a)

FIGURE 4-9 (b)

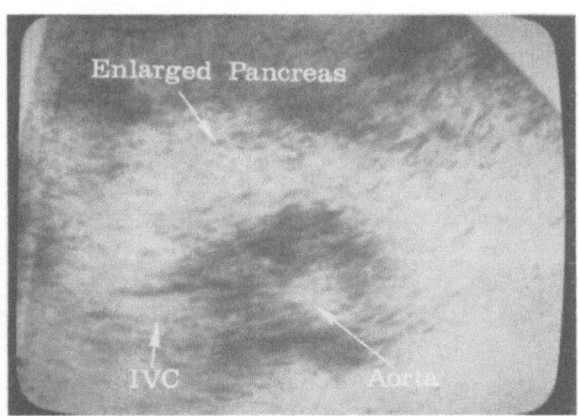

FIGURE 4.8 (b)
Supine longitudinal scan. Below the fluid-filled stomach is the echo-free enlarged pancreas. The anterior and posterior walls are well demarcated. Note the dilated superior mesenteric vein caudal to the inflamed pancreas.

FIGURE 4.9 (a)
Supine transverse scan. Magnification study. The mass over the aorta is an enlarged pancreas due to chronic inflammation. The lesion is echo-poor but transonic.

FIGURE 4.9 (b)
Supine longitudinal scan. Enlarged transonic pancreas from chronic pancreatitis. The superior mesenteric vein is dilated due to extrinsic compression by the pancreatic gland.

scan is the angled subcostal view. The margin of the inflamed pancreas is smooth and the gland becomes highly transonic (Fig. 4.8a and b).

Some investigators believe they can evaluate the enlarged pancreas of acute pancreatitis since the inflamed organ is usually separated from others in the retroperitoneum (75). The report of other authors (16) states that the phenomenon of separation is due to the sonolucency of edema. These sonographers state they cannot differentiate acute from chronic pancreatitis with acute exacerbation but are able to follow the progression or regression of the disease with sequential studies. We have noted that turgescence of the superior mesenteric vein frequently accompanies pancreatic enlargement. (Fig. 4.9a and b). Other studies show that inflammation of the pancreas is accompanied by increased fluid content, which permits better sound transmission and sharp definition of boundaries (51). Solid organs surrounding the pancreas are filled-in with echoes and the pancreas stands out in contrast. The enlarged head of the pancreas may be mistaken for a pseudocyst; however, it does not have the same degree of through transmission nor the sharp posterior wall of a cyst (Fig. 4.10a through d).

Some authors (43,52) feel that sonotomography is frequently inconclusive in chronic pancreatitis. However, large pancreatic stones may occasionally be demonstrated in the parenchyma of the gland, appearing as strong echoes within

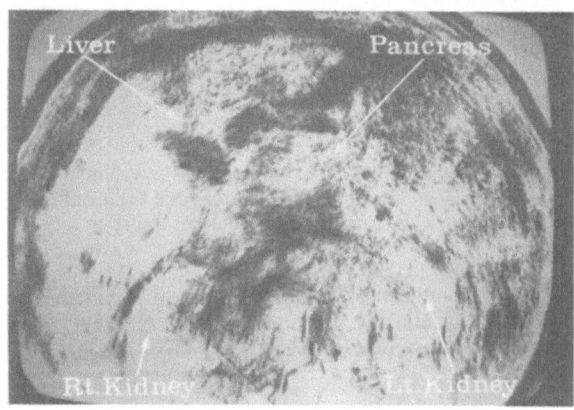

FIGURE 4-10 (a)

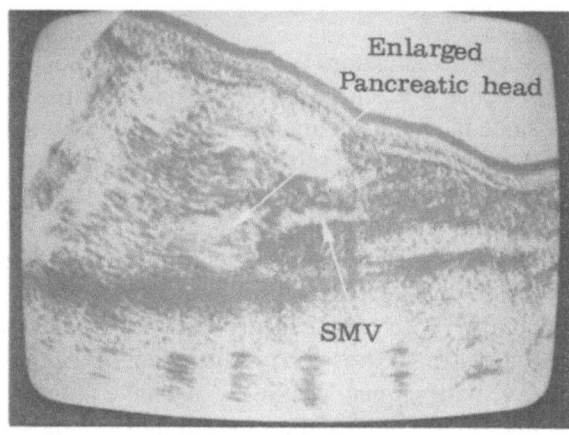

FIGURE 4-10 (b)

FIGURE 4-10 (c)

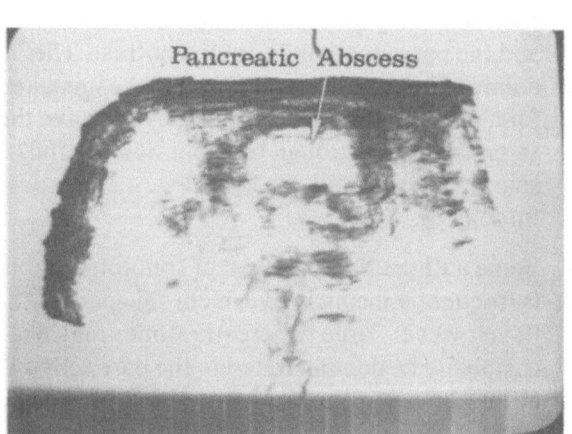

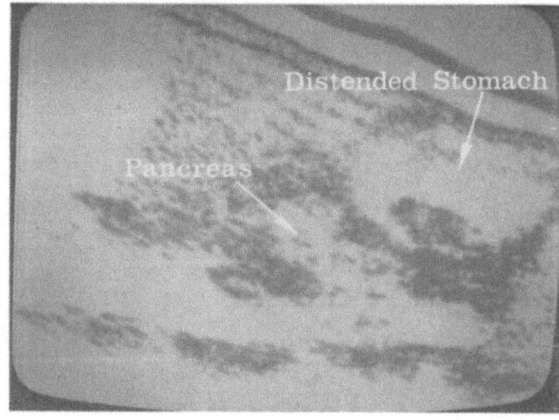

the organ indicative of chronic calculous pancreatitis. We have demonstrated the sonic shadow sign (33) in several patients with this disorder (Fig. 4.11). In chronic pancreatitis the entire gland may appear as an echogenic mass; however, delineation of the gland becomes worse as fibrosis and contraction progress.

PSEUDOCYST

Pseudocyst formation in acute pancreatitis may be demonstrated by echography as early as two weeks (51), although it usually appears eight weeks after acute inflammation. Some investigators (37,51) described the application of sonotomography in diagnosing pseudocyst of the pancreas. Their studies revealed that the pseu-

FIGURE 4.10 (a)
Supine transverse scan. Echogenic mass below the liver with a moderate degree of through transmission. The size of the enlarged pancreas due to chronic pancreatitis may be serially monitored.

FIGURE 4.10 (b)
Supine longitudinal scan. Irregular echogenic mass in the region of the head of the pancreas. Good through transmission. Chronic pancreatitis.

FIGURE 4.10 (c)
Supine transverse scan. Enlargement of the head and body of the pancreas. The area remains anechoic at high sensitivity levels. Good through transmission allows demonstration of the spine. Pancreatic abscess.

FIGURE 4.10 (d)
Supine longitudinal scan. The distended stomach reveals internal echoes from food. The distal wall of the chronically inflamed pancreas produces an echo silhouette sign at the interface with the anterior aortic wall.

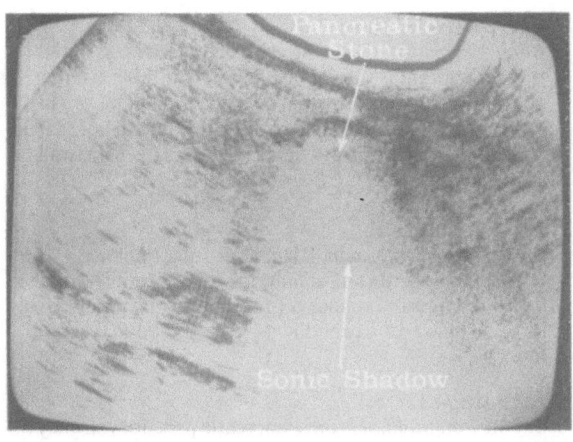

FIGURE 4.11
Supine longitudinal scan. Large pancreatic calculi may act as a specular reflector and cast a sonic shadow. Pancreatic stones indicate chronic pancreatitis.

docyst presents as a rounded sonolucent or transonic area, with a strong posterior wall echo. Our series shows these cysts may be located in any part of the pancreas and may contain septae, pus, or necrotic debris (Fig. 4.12a through d). After drainage, the cyst becomes irregular and fills-in with echoes at higher sensitivity settings.

It is stated that pseudocysts may be lobulated or multiple (16,51). We use A mode in conjunction with B-scan to prove total transonicity of the pseudocyst to differentiate it from solid tumors. The natural course of pseudocysts can be followed by sonotomography. Spontaneous rupture of a pseudocyst into the duodenum has been documented by sonography (53). The pseudocyst may resemble ascites in the region of the flank.

Other radiologic methods evaluate pseudocyst as a diagnosis of exclusion. Sonography not only directly detects the pseudocyst, but also permits temporal evaluation of this disorder.

Several entities must be included in the differential diagnosis of pancreatic pseudocyst. An enlarged gallbladder, due to carcinoma of the pancreas, must not be confused with a pseudocyst. The fluid-filled stomach may be a source of confusion. For clarification, nasogastric intubation is used to aspirate fluid from the stomach. Renal cysts of the upper pole are distinguished by prone renal scans.

Since ultrasound is atraumatic and may be safely repeated as often as necessary, we feel that sonotomography of the pancreas for pseudocyst is the diagnostic study of choice. Complications such as infection or rupture may be documented. Although complementary to angiography, sonography is superior to barium studies and isotope scans.

TUMORS

Pancreatic tumors appear as relatively echofree areas in the retroperitoneal region. Initially, the tumor is detected as a sonolucent zone; with increasing gain settings, unlike a cyst, it fills in with echoes (Fig. 4.13a and b). The shape, position, and size often vary and the

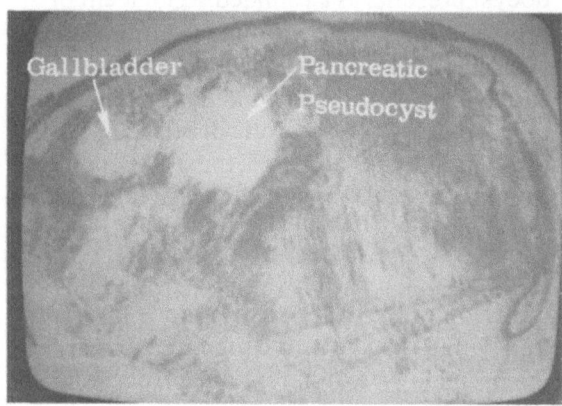

FIGURE 4-12 (a)

FIGURE 4.12 (a)
Supine transverse scan. Smooth echo-free mass in right upper quadrant is the gallbladder. To the left is a larger, less sonolucent cystic collection over the right kidney. This pancreatic pseudocyst had cloudy fluid due to internal debris, producing some low-level echoes. The distal wall is irregular.

FIGURE 4.12 (b)
Supine transverse scan. Right upper quadrant mass with cystic components and septations with irregular outlines. Scattered internal echoes represent necrotic debris in this infected pancreatic pseudocyst situated above the right kidney.

FIGURE 4.12 (c)
Supine longitudinal scan. Pancreatic pseudocysts may assume any form and vary in location. Ovoid anechoic zone above the kidney is a smooth-walled pseudocyst of the pancreas which should not be mistaken for the normal gallbladder. Transverse scanning is necessary to give a true three-dimensional representation of the cystic structure.

FIGURE 4.12 (d)
Supine transverse scan. Anechoic pancreatic pseudocyst with irregular distal wall in midline. The distended stomach has a smooth distal wall and serves as an anatomic landmark to separate the stomach from other cystic lesions.

boundary of the tumor may be smooth or irregular. It is sometimes difficult to differentiate between pancreatic tumors and other retroperitoneal space-occupying lesions.

The compressed tissue sign (16) may be present. This appears as increased echoes distal to an expanding tumor and may be caused by tissue distortion (Fig. 4.14). At the present time,

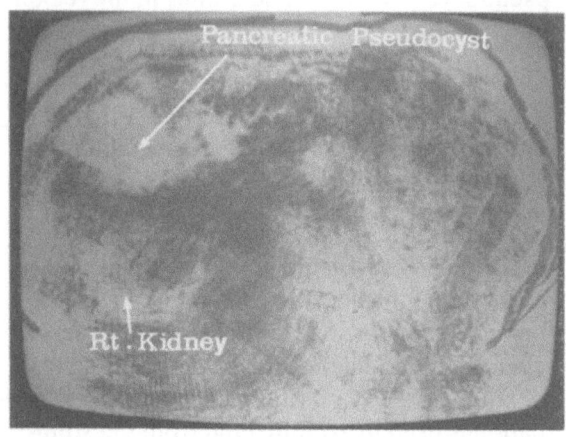

FIGURE 4-12 (b)

FIGURE 4-12 (c)

FIGURE 4-12 (d)

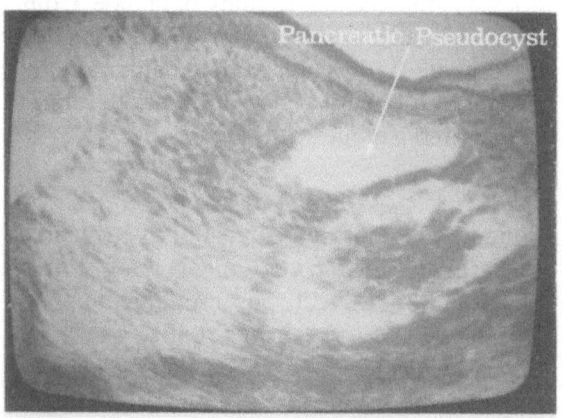

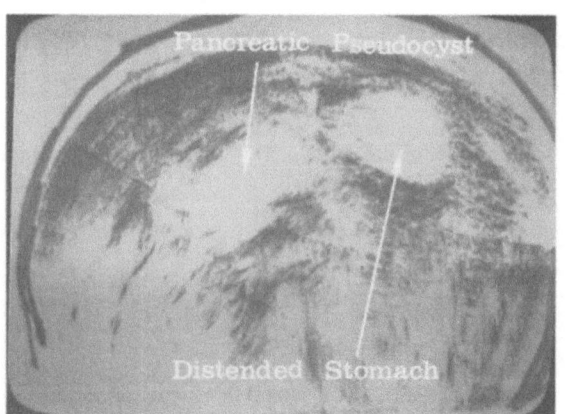

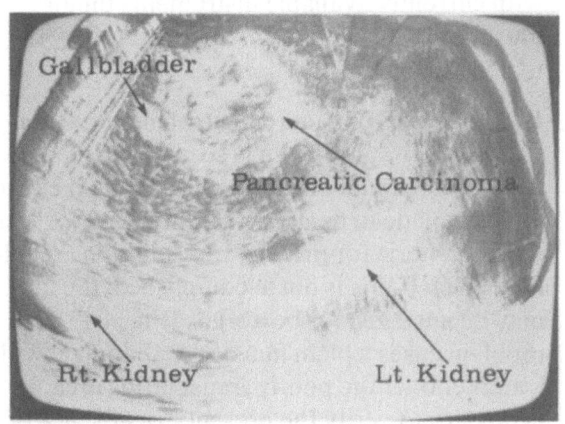

FIGURE 4.13 (a)
Supine transverse scan. Echo-free region in right upper quadrant representing neck of a dilated gallbladder. Large anechoic mass above the spine is carcinoma of the head of the pancreas. Scattered echoes represent internal degeneration.

FIGURE 4.13 (c)
Supine transverse scan. The enlarged pancreas is well circumscribed and relatively transonic. The internal echo pattern is irregular with the lighter echoes corresponding to areas of internal necrosis. Carcinoma of the head of the pancreas with dilated gallbladder.

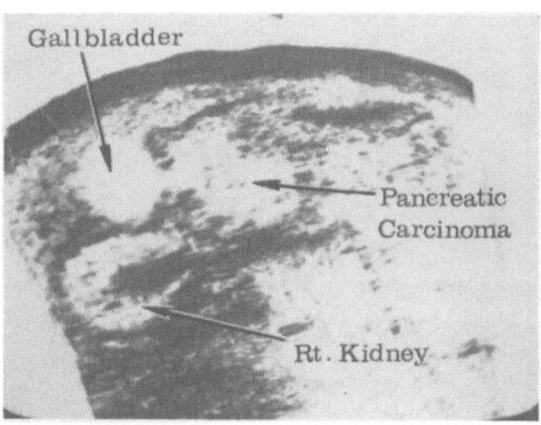

FIGURE 4.13 (b)
Supine transverse scan. Echogenic tumor mass projecting to the right of the spine. Demonstration of pancreatic carcinoma with real-time scanner. Carcinoma infiltrating the liver obliterating the hepato–pancreatic interface.

FIGURE 4.14
Supine transverse scan. The real-time scanner shows a mass between the liver and spine. The echogenic mass has produced a peripheral zone of echogenic tissue distal to it. Example of compressed tissue sign from pancreatic carcinoma.

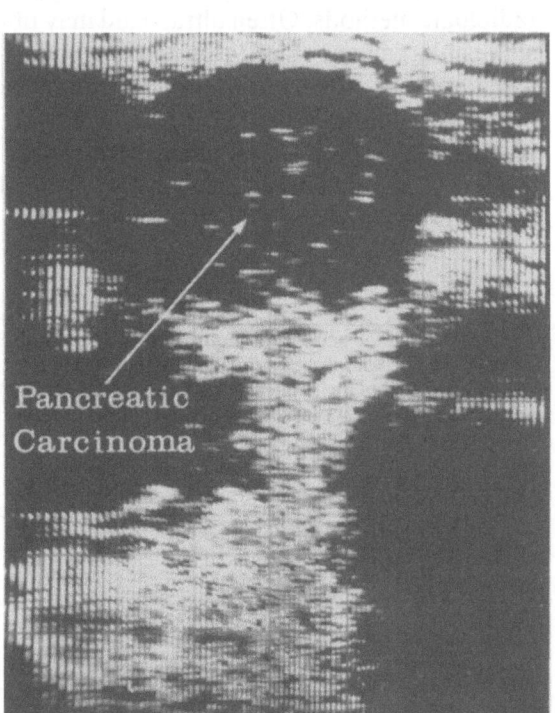

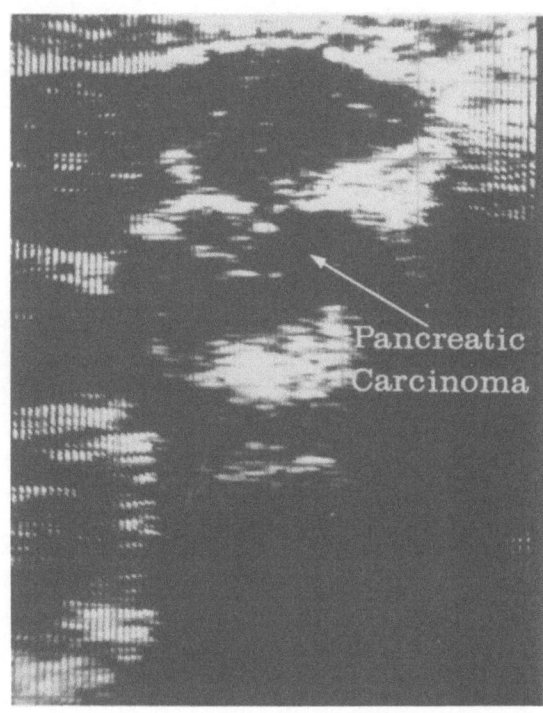

CHAPTER 4: PANCREATIC SONOGRAPHY

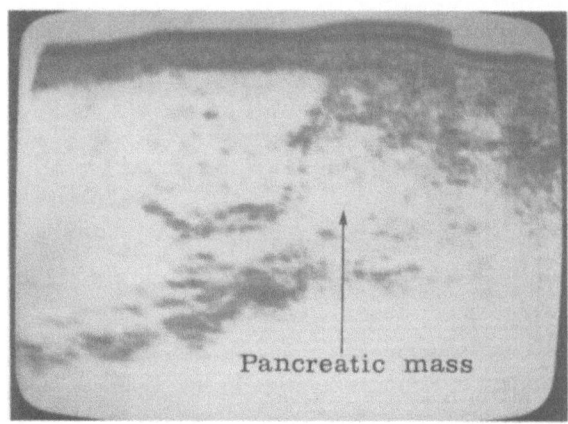

FIGURE 4-15

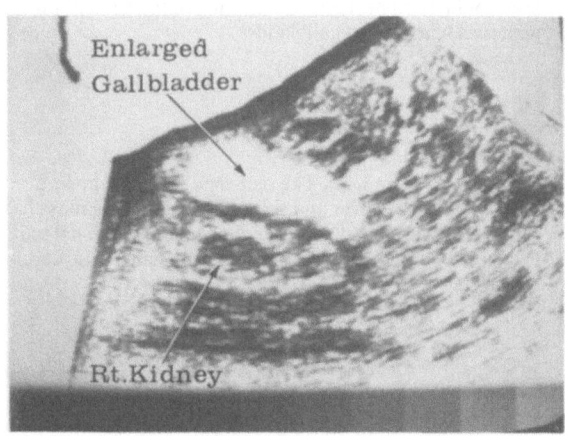

Enlarged
Gallbladder

Rt.Kidney

FIGURE 4-16 (a)

FIGURE 4-16 (b)

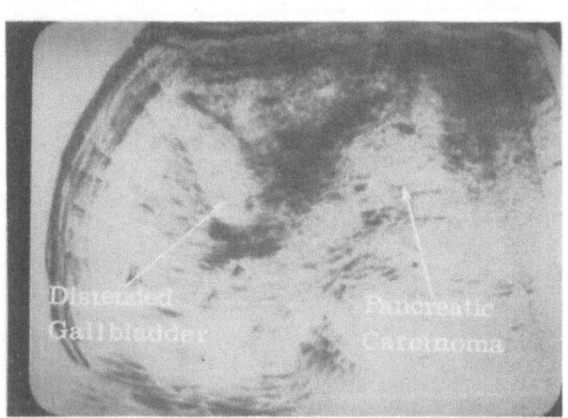

Distended
Gallbladder

Pancreatic
Carcinoma

with currently available instruments tumors must be greater than 3 cm to be accurately detected (52).

In some cases of pancreatic carcinoma, attenuation of the sonic beam is so great that the posterior wall cannot be outlined. Maximum effort must be made to demonstrate the posterior wall so that criteria for through transmission are fulfilled (31). If this is not accomplished, the tumor may be mistaken for bowel gas (Fig. 4.15). In problem cases a plain film of the abdomen, with a marker over the poorly transmitting area, is necessary to verify the presence or absence of gas to avoid misinterpretation. If there is excessive gas in the bowel, the study should be postponed.

Neoplasms generally have irregular margins and scattered internal echoes (82). Tumor in the head of the pancreas may obstruct the common bile duct, with subsequent distension of the gallbladder. An enlarged gallbladder, with a poor response to fatty meal stimulus, is one of the indirect signs of pancreatic carcinoma detectable during abdominal scanning (Fig. 4.16a and b). Carcinoma of the body and tail of the pancreas is very hard to detect by radiologic methods. Often ultrasound may observe enlargement of this area and detect the low amplitude echo pattern of a carcinoma (Fig. 4.17). Tumor obstructing the pancreatic duct may produce cystic dilatation of the duct (Fig. 4.18). Carcinoma of the pancreas may be localized or it may invade the surrounding organs

FIGURE 4.15
Supine longitudinal scan. Enormous pancreatic mass attenuating the sonic beam so that the distal wall of the mass and the anterior wall of the spine are barely imaged. This may be mistaken for the sonic shadow produced by bowel gas if maximum gain is not used.

FIGURE 4.16 (a)
Supine longitudinal scan. The enlarged gallbladder is noted overlying the kidney. There has been no change in size 1-hour post fatty meal. Note dilated cystic duct. Head is toward the right.

FIGURE 4.16 (b)
Supine transverse scan. Dilated gallbladder is noted adjacent to mass in the head of the pancreas. Pancreatic carcinoma is echo-poor.

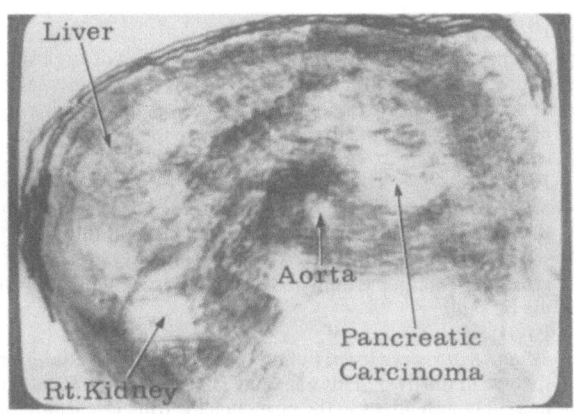

FIGURE 4-17 (a)

diffusely (Fig. 4.19). Large tumors of the pancreas may develop areas of cystic degeneration. (Fig. 4.20). Carcinoma of the ampulla of Vater or common bile duct may simulate a pancreatic neoplasm. Metastatic tumor may not be differentiated from primary carcinoma of the pancreas. This is true of malignancies originating in the vicinity of the pancreas (Fig. 4.21) and invading the organ, such as gastric and colon carcinoma or lymphoma (16). In our acoustic laboratory we periodically reevaluate patients to assess their response to chemotherapy.

Other associated pathologic conditions to be investigated are ascites (free or loculated) and

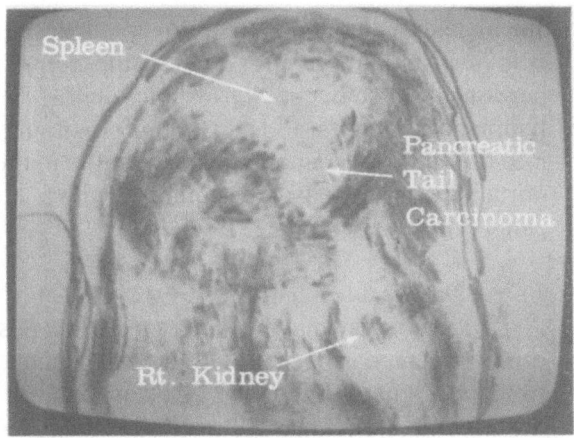

FIGURE 4-17 (b)

FIGURE 4-18

FIGURE 4.17   (a)
Supine transverse scan. Echo-poor mass in the left upper quadrant. This fairly well outlined tumor represents a slowly growing carcinoma of the tail of the pancreas with extension into the body of the gland.

FIGURE 4.17   (b)
Left lateral decubitus scan. There is a bulging mass of tissue in the splenic hilum which is indistinguishable from the spleen. Tumoris anterior to left kidney. Carcinoma tail of pancreas.

FIGURE 4.18
Supine longitudinal scan. Echo-free zone between the liver and inferior vena cava. This originates from the body of. the pancreas and represents cystic dilatation of the obstructed pancreatic duct due to carcinoma of the head of the pancreas.

FIGURE 4.19
Supine transverse scan. Massive echogenic tumor of the pancreas. The carcinoma is diffusely infiltrating the surrounding organs and the margins are poorly defined. Note the slightly enlarged gallbladder.

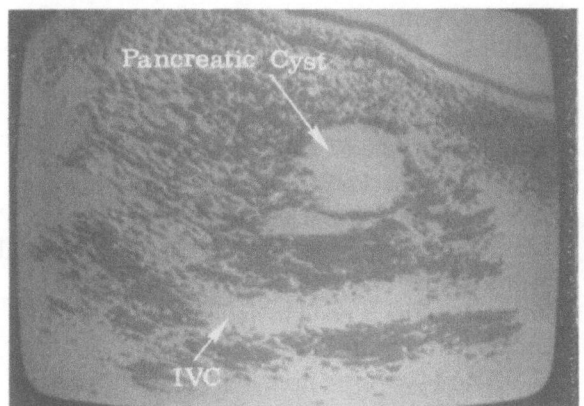

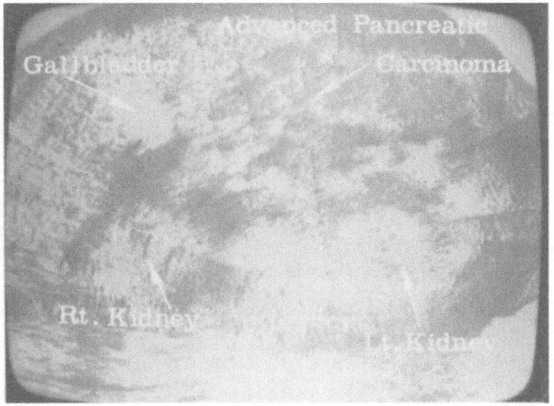

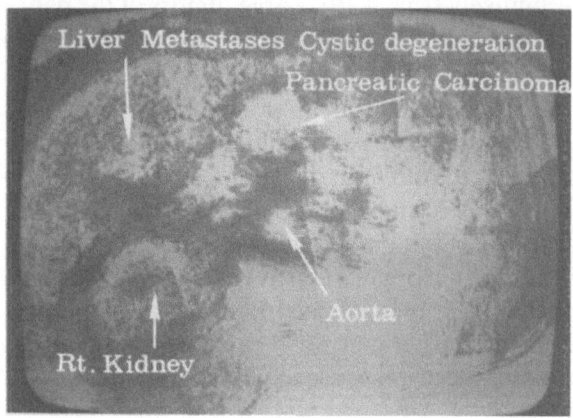

FIGURE 4-20

FIGURE 4.20
Supine transverse scan. Pancreatic carcinoma of large size with echo-free central region representing cystic internal degeneration of the tumor. This may be confused with a pseudocyst. Note the irregular anechoic foci of metastatic lesions in the liver.
FIGURE 4.21
Supine transverse scan. A large echogenic mass is noted in the anterior simulating a pancreatic neoplasm. Multiple sonolucent regions are noted distant from this mass and represent enlarged lymph nodes in this case of lymphoma of the mesentery.
FIGURE 4.22
Supine transverse scan. Echo-poor mass below the inferior surface of the liver. This anechoic sheet of tumor represents matted lymph nodes in the porta hepatis from metastatic carcinoma.

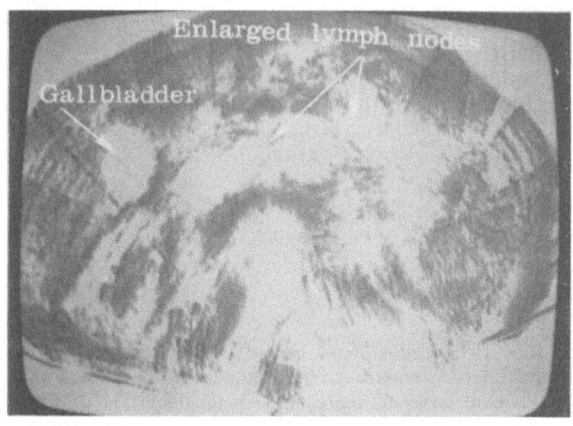

FIGURE 4-21

FIGURE 4-22

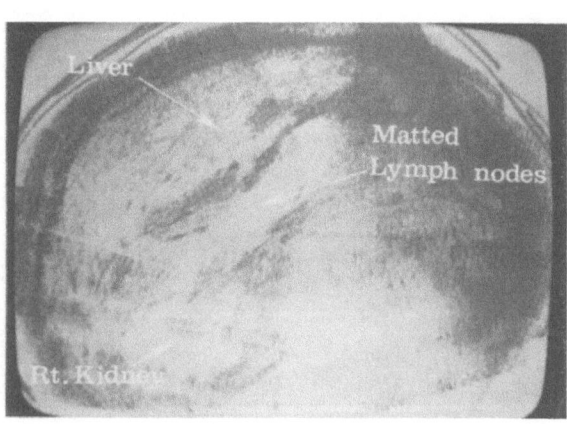

splenic enlargement due to portal or splenic vein obstruction. The presence of other retroperitoneal space-occupying lesions, such as lymph node masses, adds further information into the study. Indeed, lymphadenopathy in the porta hepatis may easily be confused with a pancreatic mass (Fig. 4.22).

Percutaneous fine needle biopsy
Aspiration biopsy may be performed when it is otherwise impossible to differentiate a benign from a malignant lesion (30). A lesion may be demonstrated on cross-sectional scan if it is 3 cm (52). The special tunnel transducer is used. The puncture needle is introduced through the tunnel, following the direction of the sonic beam. The depth to the desired area is read from the oscilloscope. The patient is in the supine position and the hilus of the right kidney is located. With multiple oblique sections, the pancreas is delineated. The best landmarks for the pancreas are the aorta, inferior vena cava, and posterior side of the left lobe of liver. The left kidney, spleen, and portal vein, and, if possible, the superior mesenteric artery are also useful. It is good practice to identify the gallbladder by shape and the duodenum by peristaltic movement. For stomach localization, a nasogastric tube is used to aspirate air. Then 100 ml of gasless water is introduced and the scan then shows a cystic area in front of the pancreas. By this method, the tumor and organs in the

vicinity of the lesion are identified and the optimal site for puncture is marked over the skin. After the skin is sterilized and infiltrated with a local anesthetic, the scan is repeated with a tunnel transducer, aiming the sonic beam toward the area of interest. A guide cannula, 1 to 2 mm in outer diameter, is introduced through the transducer. A fine needle, with an outer diameter of 0.6 mm, is then introduced through the cannula. The depth of the lesion is determined from the oscilloscope and is marked on the fine needle.

Aspiration is performed using suction on the syringe attached to the needle. Routinely, four to six punctures in various directions are performed through the same guide cannula passed through the liver. The biopsy is taken in suspended respiration. The patient should be fasting.

Prior to biopsy, the patient should be evaluated for hemorrhagic diathesis. The material obtained is smeared on a slide, fixed in methyl alcohol for five minutes, and stained by the Giemsa method. Spread of tumor cells is negligible with the fine needle biopsy method (30). Surgery is usually indicated in the presence of obstructive jaundice. However, a laparotomy may be avoided in the patient with an incurable tumor, but without cholestasis.

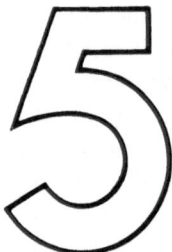

vascular sonography

ABDOMINAL AORTA

SONOGRAPHY

The investigation of pulsatile abdominal masses presents special problems. Most of these masses represent extreme tortuousity of the distal abdominal aorta (68). However, clinical differentiation from a true aortic aneurysm may be difficult (74).

Sonography is not only an excellent diagnostic modality but also the least invasive for the detection and follow-up of aortic aneurysms. Indeed, this was one of the first uses of ultrasound in the upper abdomen. Improved diagnostic techniques have revealed a greater incidence of asymptomatic abdominal aortic aneurysms in the elderly than was previously recognized (29,74).

Abdominal aortic ultrasonography assumes increased importance since this may be the only method available for examining the geriatric patient.

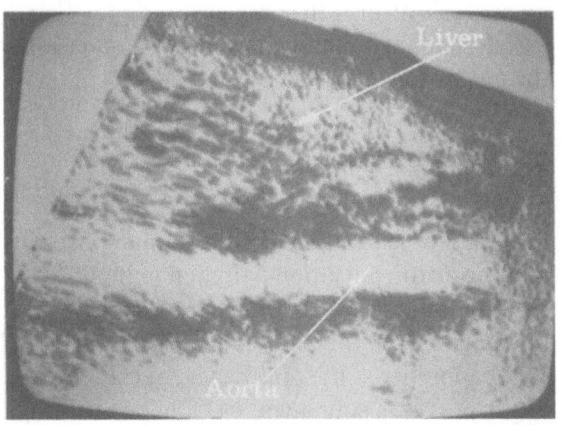

FIGURE 5.1 (a)
Supine longitudinal scan. The aorta appears as a linear echo-free structure that tapers smoothly. It may usually be imaged from the xiphoid process down to the level of the umbilicus. Usually the distal wall is more sharply outlined than the proximal wall. The origin of the superior mesenteric artery may often be visualized anterior to the aorta.

FIGURE 5.1 (b)
Supine longitudinal scan. The aorta may be easily studied with the real-time scanner. The characteristic systolic contraction wave may be observed. This verifies the aorta and distinguishes it from other echo-free regional structures.

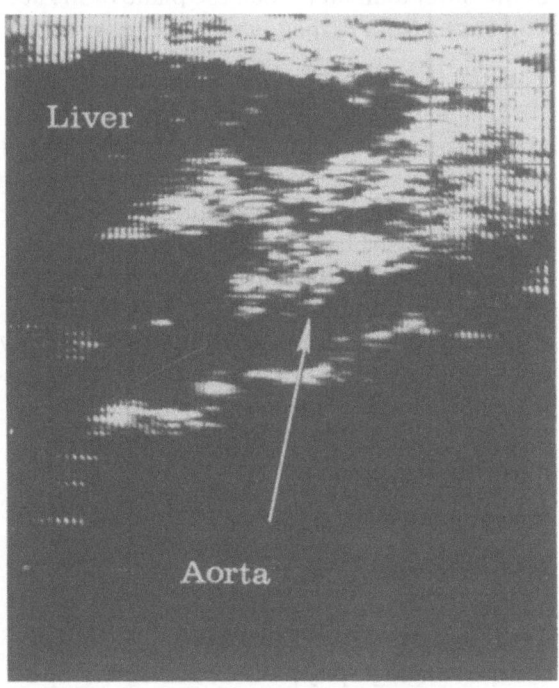

ANATOMY

The abdominal aorta begins at the aortic hiatus in the diaphragm in front of the lower border of the twelfth dorsal vertebral body. It descends anterior to the vertebral column and ends at the bifurcation into the iliac arteries at the fourth lumbar vertebra.

Anterior and proximally, the celiac and superior mesenteric arteries arise from the aorta. Below this area the left renal vein and the body of the pancreas, with its posterior splenic vein, cross obliquely. Below the level of the second lumbar vertebra the inferior vena cava is located to the right of the aorta. On the left side of the aorta are the duodenojejunal flexure, ascending duodenum, and visceral arteries.

The normal aorta in thin patients is very close to the anterior abdominal wall.

SONOANATOMY

Blood is a good transonic medium. Consequently, the aorta can be easily detected by abdominal sonolaparotomy (Fig. 5.1a and b).

The aorta is located anterior to the spine, generally slightly to the left. Its walls reflect strong echoes, with an anechoic region representing the blood-containing lumen. The caliber of the normal aorta is approximately 3 cm and it tapers off as it descends. On gray scale, blood does not have the same homogeneity as clear fluid.

There is no magnification, and the size of the aorta may be accurately determined. Simple measurement may be accomplished by calculating the anterior to posterior diameter in the longitudinal or transverse sections.

Transverse, longitudinal, and even occasionally oblique views are necessary to detect aortic pathology. The study is made easier by applying the real-time scanner and gray scale. With the real-time scanner, the course of the superior mesenteric vein can be followed to the junction of the portal vein, and the superior mesenteric vein can be differentiated from the superior

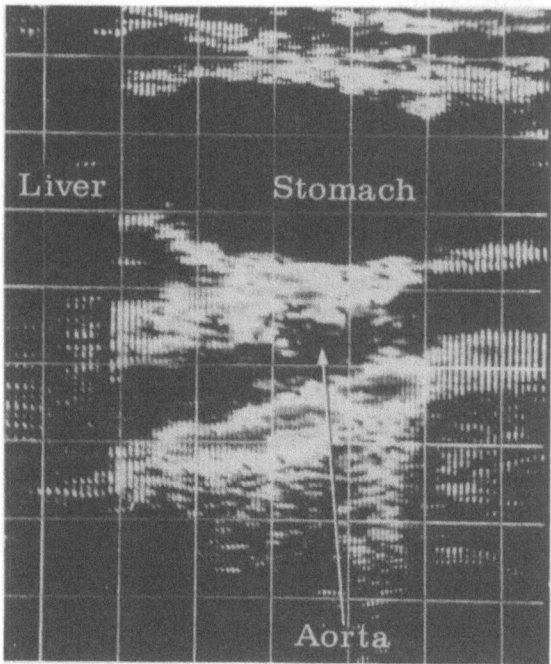

FIGURE 5.2
Supine longitudinal scan. In difficult cases with overlying
bowel gas, the stomach may be distended with fluid, creating a sonic window caudal to the liver edge. The abdominal
aorta is the tubular echo-free structure distal to the ovoid
anechoic lumen of the stomach imaged with the real-time
scanner.

FIGURE 5.3
Supine longitudinal scan. An abrupt termination of the
aortic lumen is frequently seen, with aortic tortuousity
when the vessel passes out of the plane of the scan. Embol-
us or thrombosis may produce a similar picture.

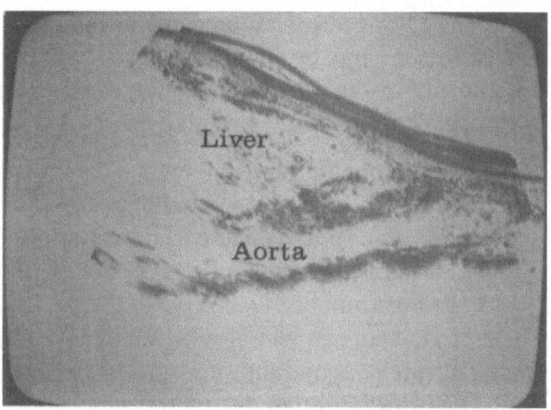

mesenteric artery. In some cases, distending
the stomach with fluid simplifies examination of
the aorta (Fig. 5.2).

SONOLAPAROTOMY

The patient is examined in the supine position
and the aortic pulsation palpated manually before scanning. The abdominal aorta can usually
be imaged from the xiphoid process to the level
of the umbilicus. In some cases, overlying bowel gas prevents sound waves from penetrating.
In rescanning, the examiner should try to displace the gas by manual palpation, otherwise,
the study must be postponed. The abdomen is
initially scanned longitudinally to observe the
course and tortuousity of the aorta in the sagit-
tal plane. Sudden discontinuity in the course of
the abdominal aorta is either due to tortuousity
(Fig. 5.3) or occlusion. It is good practice to
mark the path of the previously palpated, maximum pulsation of the aorta on the skin. Both
the anterior and posterior walls must be visualized.

B-scan cross-sections are then made at right
angles to the aorta to prevent misrepresentation
of the outer diameter when the plane of the section varies from perpendicular to the vessel.

The lumen can be identified more readily if the
aorta is imaged by gray scale (Fig. 5.1a) and
magnification studies may be performed for better evaluation. The real-time scanner demonstrates the aorta clearly and pulsation of its
walls can be displayed on the television monitor. Occasionally, the aorta can be demonstrated more accurately if the stomach is distended
with fluid (Fig. 5.2). By changing the sensitivity
of the real-time scanner, the nature of the pulsations can be better imaged and pathologic conditions, such as asynchrony of the walls, are
more easily determined.

SONOPATHOLOGY

Traditionally, the aorta has been studied with
contrast angiography by the translumbar ap-

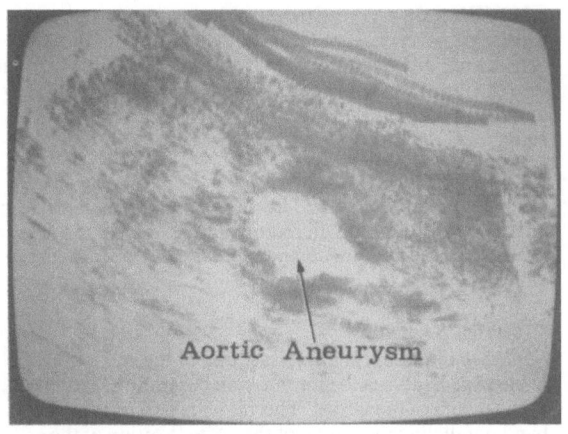

FIGURE 5.4
Supine longitudinal scan. Aneurysm of the aorta may be confused with other cystic structures. The entrance of the aorta into the dilatation and its exit from the aneurysmal sac are important in definitively diagnosing a saccular abdominal aortic aneurysm.

FIGURE 5.5
Supine longitudinal scan. The distal aortic walls become a fusiform aneurysm. At low sensitivity, the outer walls are clearly demonstrated. At higher-gain settings, the thrombus within the lumen will be demonstrated as low-amplitude echoes.

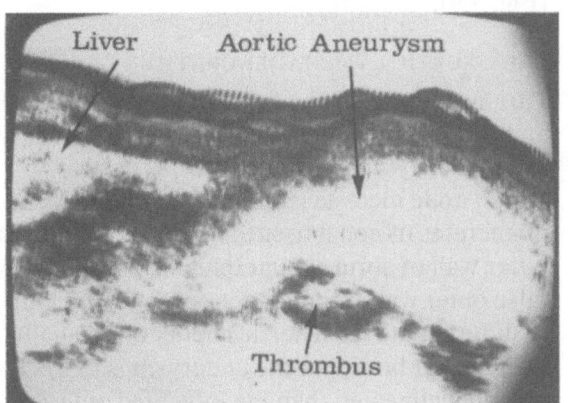

proach or through percutaneous, retrograde, femoral artery catheterization. However, serious consequences may accompany these methods. A known incidence of thrombosis and embolization is associated with arterial catheterization, especially after a plaque, in patients with severe atherosclerosis is punctured. Since systemic hypertension is frequently associated with atherosclerosis, hematomas may form at the puncture site.

ANEURYSM

Arteriography can only show the patient lumen of an aneurysm; the clotted portion obviously cannot be seen. The true size of an aneurysm is assessed by measuring the width of the lumen on the angiogram and adding to it the distance from the lumen to the outer calcified wall. If calcification can not be seen radiologically, the true dimensions of the aneurysm cannot be accurately estimated. In fact, if there is no wall calcification and the laminated thrombus completely fills the aneurysmal sac, the contrast-opacified lumen of the aortic aneurysm may be mistaken for a normal distal aorta and the diagnosis completely missed (68,73). The outer diameter is an important preoperative parameter for the surgeon. Elective operation is considered when this measurement exceeds 7 cm (23,73,74).

Abdominal aortic aneurysms may assume a variety of forms. Dilatation may be localized and the aneurysm saccular shaped. It usually has a sharp anterior wall, and may easily be confused with a cystic lesion. However, the outer wall of a cyst is generally not as sharp as that of an aneurysm (Fig. 5.4). Fusiform aneurysms typically start below the level of the renal arteries in the region of the inferior border of the liver but they may involve the entire abdominal aorta (Fig. 5.5). Fusiform aneurysms may extend into the iliac arteries (Fig. 5.6), and may involve long segments of the aorta, beginning in the thoracic aorta and extending into the abdominal aorta. This thoracoabdominal aneurysm appears on the abdominal scan as dilated lumen that tapers in size as it descends into the lower abdomen (Fig. 5.7).

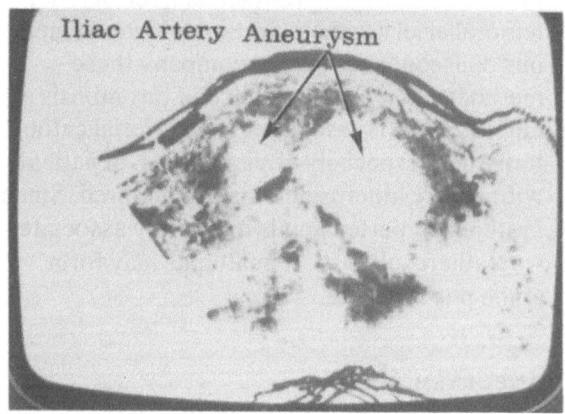

FIGURE 5-6

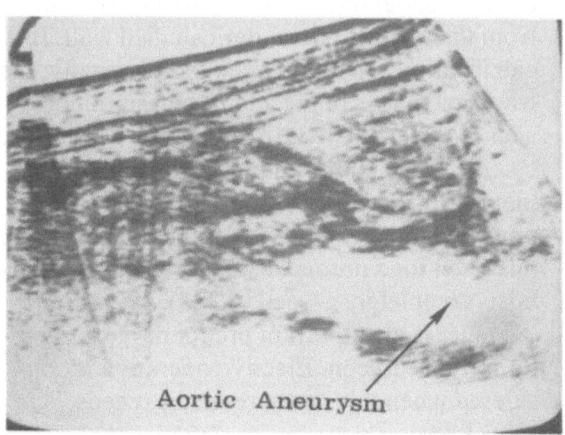

FIGURE 5-7

FIGURE 5-8 (a)

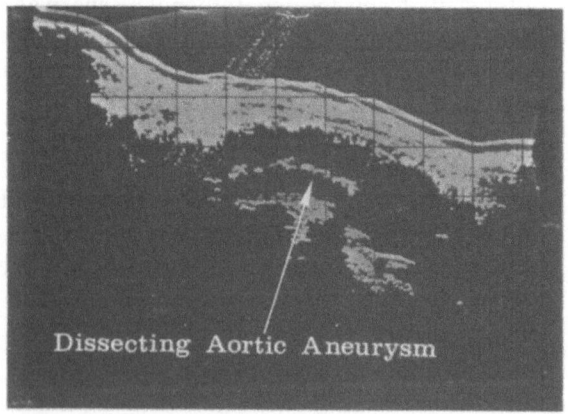

FIGURE 5.6
FIGURE 5.6
Supine transverse scan. Echo-free dilatations of the iliac arteries are demonstrated. Extension of an aortic aneurysm into the iliac vessels is not uncommon. The left iliac artery aneurysm is larger than the aneurysmal dilatation on the right.

FIGURE 5.7
Supine longitudinal scan. The thoracoabdominal aortic aneurysm appears as a dilatation of the lumen of the aorta at the level of the diaphragm and tapers to the normal aortic caliber. Head is toward the right.

FIGURE 5.8 (a)
Supine longitudinal scan. Dissection of the wall of the aneurysm displaces the intimal wall centrally as blood runs in the media of the vessel. This appears as a linear echo band paralleling the lumen of the aorta. Motion of the intimal wall may be observed with M-mode or real-time scanner.

Various layers of the aneurysm can be detected by adjusting the sensitivity of the ultrasonic unit. At low sensitivity, only the outer walls of the aneurysm are seen. Higher sensitivity will show echoes from the clot or thrombus (Fig. 5.5). The true lumen, filled with blood, remains echo free.

Dissecting aneurysm occurs less often in the abdominal than the thoracic aorta. Intimal necrosis permits blood to course in the media of the vessel. External rupture may occur or the channel may reenter the aortic lumen. The intima is pushed into the blood-filled true lumen by the intramural hemorrhage, which appears as a septation in the echo-free aorta (Fig. 5.8a and b) generally best seen on the longitudinal scan. At higher sensitivities, the thrombus in the false channel may fill-in with echoes. Thrombus is best demonstrated with gray-scale equipment (Fig. 5.9).

PARA-AORTIC LYMPHADENOPATHY

Para-aortic lymphadenopathy occurs in benign and malignant states. Large preaortic masses are seen in lymphoma and retroperitoneal lymph node metastases (Fig. 5.10). These conglomerates of nodal tissue silhouette the normal outer wall of aorta sonographically, creating a false outer wall. Lymphadenopathy is difficult to differentiate from aortic aneurysm. Usually, the anterior border of the aneurysm is more sharply delineated than the lobulated anterior

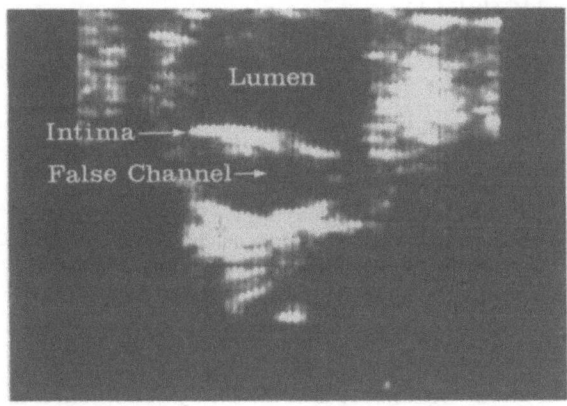

FIGURE 5-8 (b)

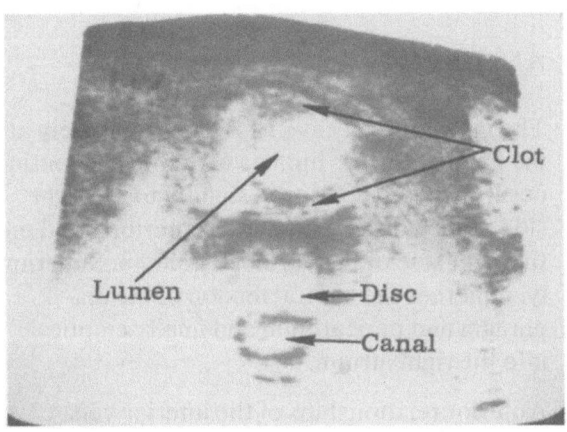

FIGURE 5-9

FIGURE 5-10

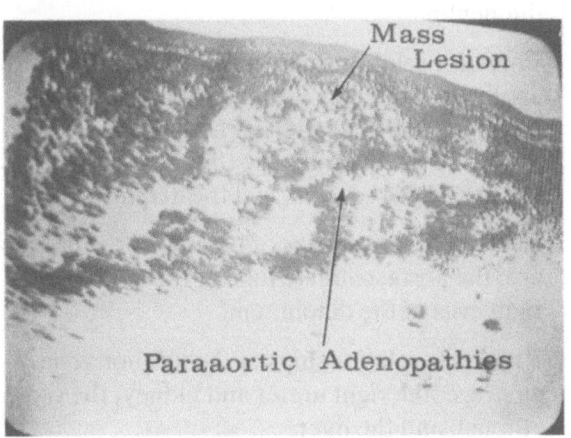

FIGURE 5.8 (b)
Supine transverse scan. The aorta is dilated to 8 cm. The sharp echogenic distal wall of the aneurysm is noted as a concave surface. A linear band of high amplitude echoes crossing transversely represents the intimal wall pushed into the lumen. Dissecting aneurysm.

FIGURE 5.9
Supine transverse scan. Three anechoic regions are noted. Anterior is an aortic aneurysm with an inner layer of thrombus producing an echo-free lumen. Distal to the aneurysm is the echo-poor intervertebral disc. Distally are noted parts of the neural arch forming the spinal canal.

FIGURE 5.10
Supine longitudinal scan. Para-aortic lymph node masses may silhouette the outline of the normal aorta creating a falsely enlarged lumen. Other regions of enlarged lymph nodes must be sought to differentiate periaortic lymphadenopathy from a true aneurysm.

border of lymph node masses (Fig. 5.10). To confirm para-aortic lymph nodes, other areas of lymphadenopathy must be sought.

A confusing artifact frequently occurs when the plane of the scanning beam passes through the fibrocartilaginous intervertebral discs of thin patients. Although the body of the vertebra blocks sonic transmission, the disc structure appears echo free at low sensitivities and may be echogenic at higher gain settings. The neural arch elements may be partly visualized, forming an outline of the spinal canal. In transverse scanning, the anechoic disc may be mistaken for a cystic or vascular structure (Fig. 5.9). This problem can be resolved by sensitivity studies and M-mode or real-time scanners.

INFERIOR VENA CAVA

SONOGRAPHY

Imaging of the inferior vena cava and simultaneous measurements of its diameter are valuable in conditions that cause this vessel to distend. The etiology of the turgescent vessel, such as right heart failure, can be determined by evaluating the dilated inferior vena cava. Hepatomegaly due to right heart failure can be diagnosed by scanning the inferior vena cava. The normal vessel collapses during the expiratory phase of respiration but does not do so in the

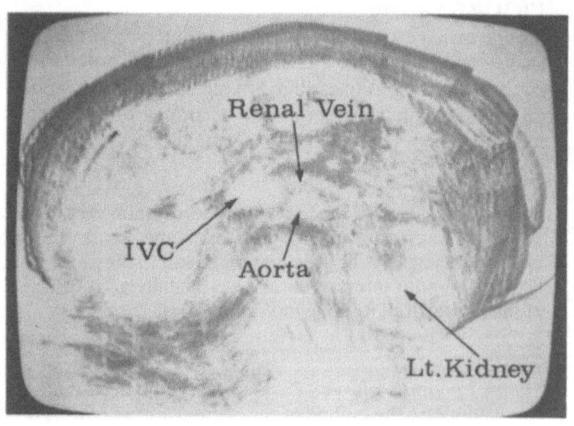

FIGURE 5-11

FIGURE 5.11
Supine transverse scan. The left renal vein is longer than the right and crosses over the aorta to join the inferior vena cava.

FIGURE 5.12 (a)
Supine longitudinal scan. The superior mesenteric vein is noted above the inferior vena cava. It normally dilates at the junction with the splenic vein to form the portal vein. The superior mesenteric vein is much larger than the superior mesenteric artery. This distinction may be made with gray-scale scanning.

patient with heart failure. This phenomenon is best studied with the real-time scanner.

Inferior vena cava imaging can also be used to detect a thrombus or tumor in this structure.

ANATOMY

The inferior vena cava starts approximately at the level of the 5th lumbar vertebra and continues its course superiorly, slightly to the right side of the aorta. It is located anteriorly and on the right side of the vertebral column. Superiorly, it pierces the central tendon of the diaphragm and pericardium and finally empties into the right atrium.

Anterior relationships of the inferior vena cava are (caudal to cephalad) the right common iliac artery, the root of the mesentery and peritoneum, the right testicular or ovarian vessels, the third part of the duodenum and the head of the pancreas, the gastroduodenal artery, the bile duct, the portal vein, and the first part of the duodenum.

Posterior relationships of the inferior vena cava are (caudal to cephalad) the psoas major, the lumbar artery, the anterior longitudinal ligament, the lower lumbar vertebrae, the renal artery, the right adrenal, and the diaphragm.

Left side relationships of the inferior vena cava are: the aorta, caudate lobe of the liver, and right crus of the diaphragm.

Right side relationships of the inferior vena cava are: the right ureter and kidney, the right adrenal, and the liver.

FIGURE 5-12 (a)

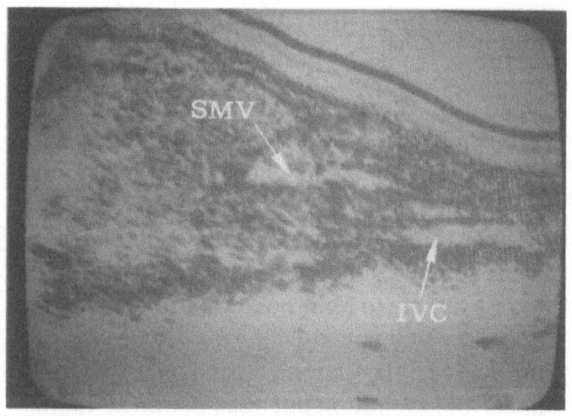

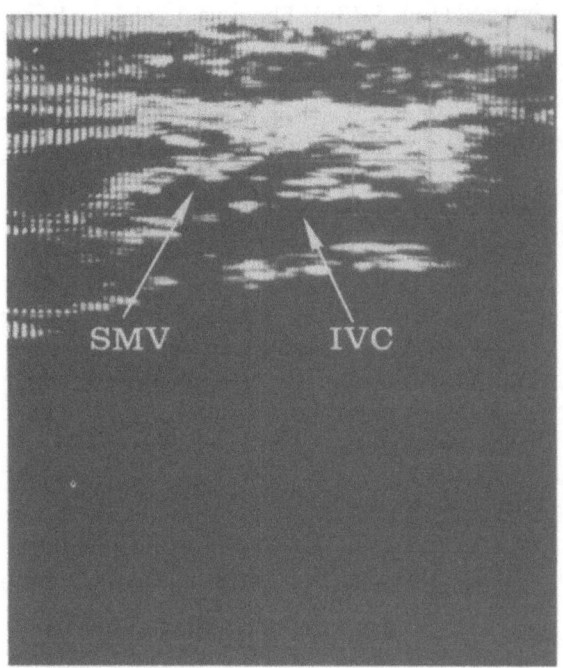

FIGURE 5-12 (b)

FIGURE 5.12 (b)
Supine longitudinal scan. Sonofluoroscopy with the real-time scanner demonstrates the tubular outline of the inferior vena cava with its phasic respiratory changes. Above this is the superior mesenteric vein.

FIGURE 5.12 (c)
Supine longitudinal scan. Fast scanning speed over the inverior vena cava may demonstrate a wavy outline to this vessel due to inherent motion.

The inferior vena cava, in its upward course, reaches to a much higher vertebral level than does the aorta. In its uppermost portion, the inferior vena cava is partially embedded in the liver. Consequently, it is extremely important to detect the inferior vena cava in this area, because the liver covers it not only anteriorly, but also extends to both the right and left sides of the vein. The inferior vena cava terminates at the level of the 8th thoracic vertebra and the 6th costal cartilage. The left renal vein has a longer course and passes over the aorta to empty into the inferior vena cava (Fig. 5.11). The right renal vein is not as long and is extremely hard to visualize in the normal individual.

SONONANATOMY

The image of the inferior vena cava in longitudinal section is usually very difficult to visualize when the scan is performed with conventional equipment, but is easy to demonstrate by real-time scanner and gray scale (Fig. 5.12a, b, and c). In a normal subject, during inspiration the vena cava reaches maximum diameter after a few seconds. At least several seconds are required to produce this image when a manual probe is used. During this interval, the size of the inferior vena cava changes and it is blurred in the longitudinal section.

If the examination has been done in the Valsalva maneuver, sufficient delay allows the inferior vena cava to be well visualized. In cross-sectional studies, the inferior vena cava and its relation with the aorta, superior mesenteric artery and superior mesenteric vein can usually be

FIGURE 5-12 (c)

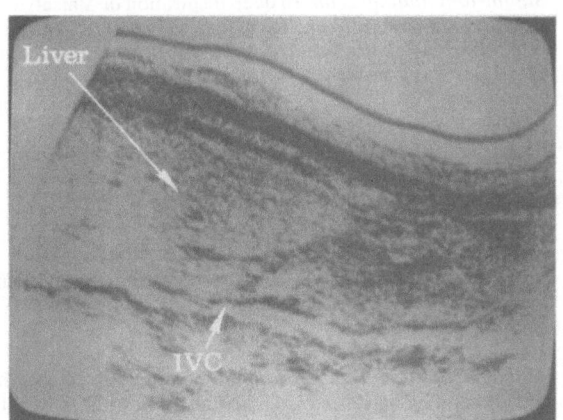

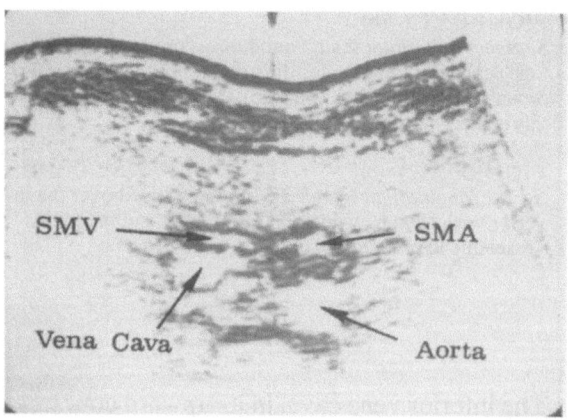

FIGURE 5-13 (a)

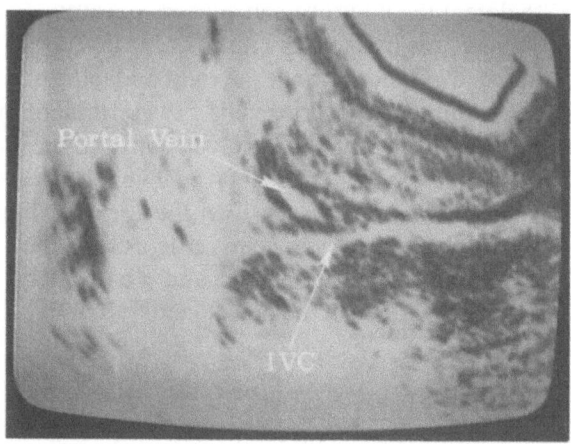

FIGURE 5-13 (b)

FIGURE 5-13 (c)

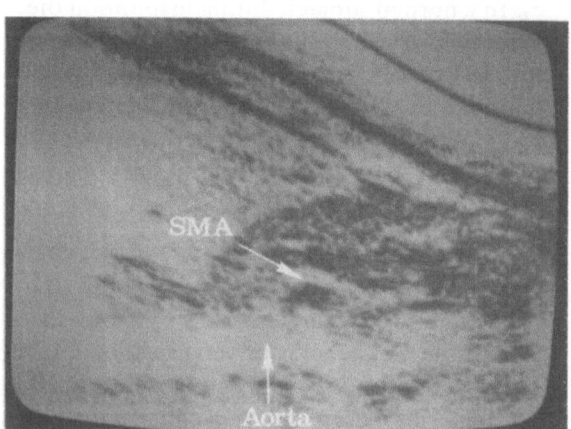

imaged (Fig. 5.13a). The portal vein can be imaged in longitudinal scans (Fig. 5.13b), and the superior mesenteric artery seen over the aorta or vena cava (Fig. 5.13c). The study performed with the real-time scanner in the paramedian approach shows the vessel's complex motion, which corresponds to the respiratory cycle. The liver and aorta transmit systolic pressure to the inferior vena cava so that the anterior wall of the vein has even more intense motion than the anterior wall of the aorta (83). During inspiration, it is well filled and prominent; during expiration it is collapsed and not easily visualized (Fig. 5.14a, b, and c).

SHIFTING METHOD

Where uncertainty exists in verification of the inferior vena cava, the aorta can easily be found

FIGURE 5.13 (a)
Supine transverse scan. The echo-free aorta and inferior vena cava are adjacent. Above the inferior vena cava is the flattened superior mesenteric vein. Above the aorta is the superior mesenteric artery.

FIGURE 5.13 (b)
Supine longitudinal scan. The elliptical shaped portal vein is seen above the inferior vena cava.

FIGURE 5.13 (c)
Supine longitudinal scan. The origin of the superior mesenteric artery from the aorta is well demonstrated. This artery then runs parallel to the aorta.

FIGURE 5.14 (a)
Supine longitudinal scan. The echo-free tubular inferior vena cava in normal respiration. The portal vein is partially imaged. Head is toward the right.

FIGURE 5.14 (b)
Supine longitudinal scan. In deep inspiration or Valsalva maneuver the inferior vena cava dilates. The portal vein lying anterior to the inferior vena cava is better appreciated. Head is toward the right.

FIGURE 5.14 (c)
Supine longitudinal scan. The distal inferior vena cava is collapsed in deep expiration. This is a normal respiratory phenomenon. Head is toward the right.

FIGURE 5.15 (a)
Supine longitudinal scan. The inferior vena cava is easily visualized with the real time scanner.

FIGURE 5.15 (b)
Supine longitudinal scan. From this anatomic structure, the applicator may be shifted to locate the aorta with its systolic contractions.

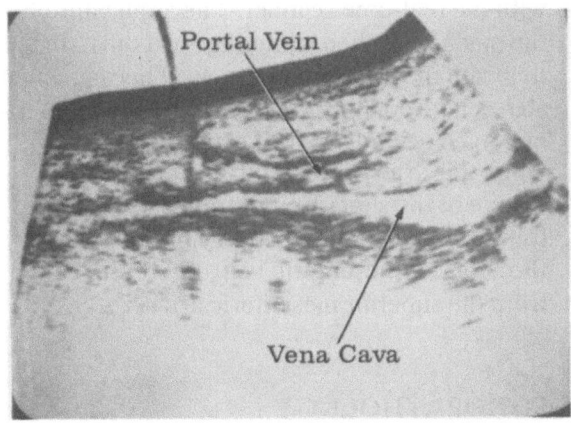

FIGURE 5-14 (a)

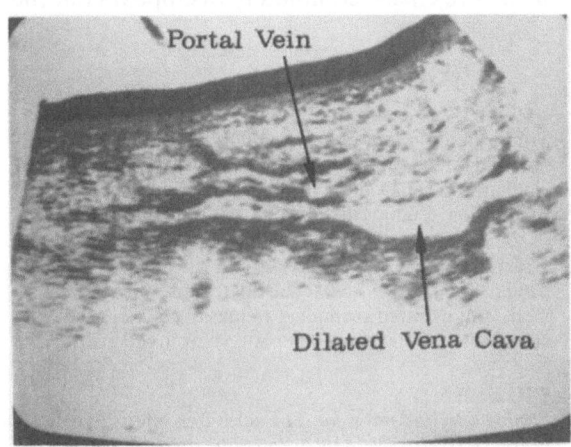

FIGURE 5-14 (b)

FIGURE 5-14 (c)

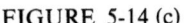
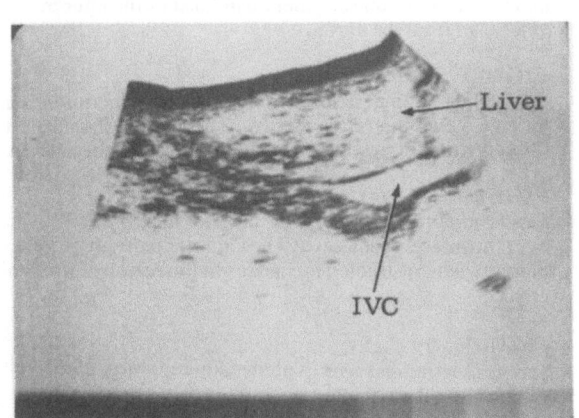

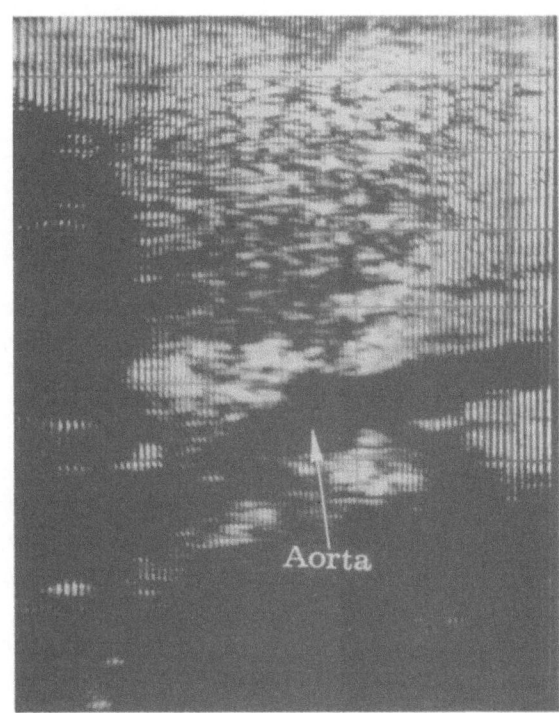

FIGURE 5-15 (a)

FIGURE 5-15 (b)

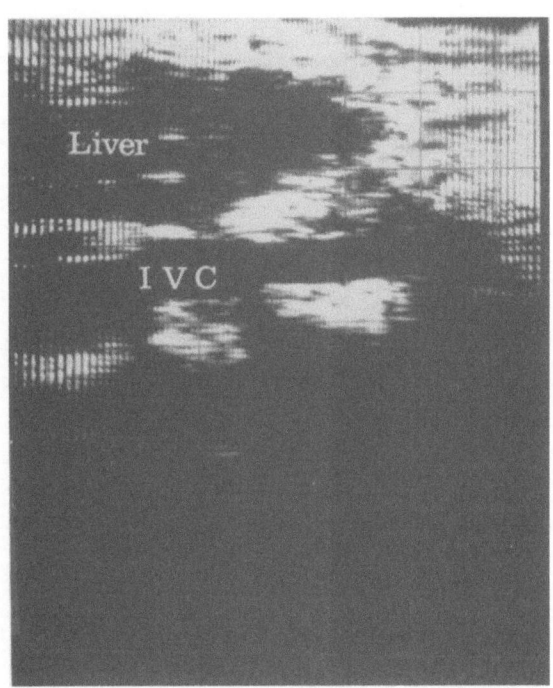

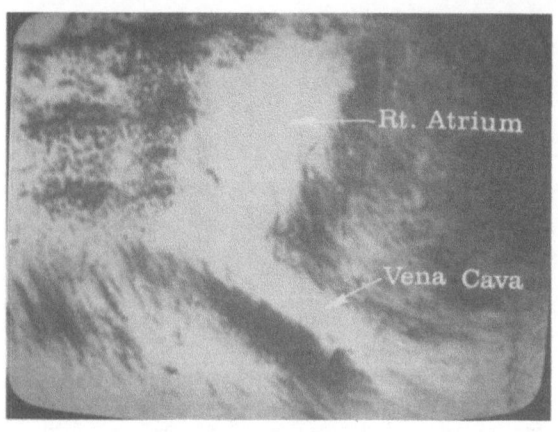

FIGURE 5-16 (a)

FIGURE 5-16 (b)

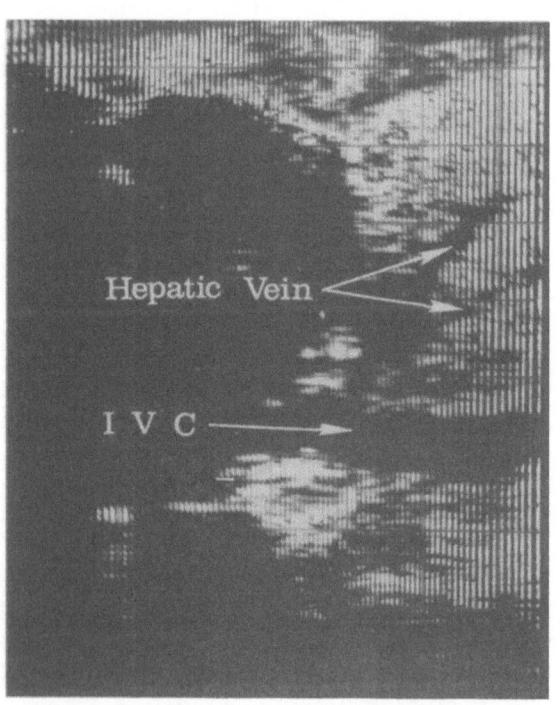

with the real-time scanner. The applicator of the machine is then shifted toward the right side to locate the inferior vena cava. This maneuver also can be done from the location of the inferior vena cava toward the aorta (Fig. 5.15a, b), when this artery is difficult to identify. The course of the superior mesenteric vein can be followed to the junction of the portal vein and the superior mesenteric vein differentiated from the superior mesenteric artery.

SONOPATHOLOGY

In right-sided cardiac conditions, the respiratory motion of the vena cava diminishes and, in severe cases, completely disappears but the

FIGURE 5.16　(a)
Supine longitudinal scan. The dilated inferior vena cava is situated on the right side of the midline and passes into the right atrium. The caliber of this vessel did not change with respiration. Venous distension from right heart failure.

FIGURE 5.16　(b)
Supine longitudinal scan. The dilated inferior vena cava well demonstrated secondary to massive pericardial effusion. Note tubular dilated hepatic veins in the liver.

FIGURE 5.17
Supine longitudinal scan. The echo-free inferior vena cava is anteriorly displaced by an anechoic mass of clustered lymph nodes.

FIGURE 5.18
Supine longitudinal scan. The posteriorly displaced aorta may simulate a dilated inferior vena cava that has been pushed by a mass. The inferior vena cava usually collapses at the point of compression while the aortic lumen remains patent. The real-time scanner distinguishes the inferior vena cava from the aorta.

FIGURE 5.19　(a)
Supine longitudinal scan. Echo-free dilated superior mesenteric vein over inferior vena cava. This finding should alert the sonographer to study the pancreatic region for masses.

FIGURE 5.19　(b)
Supine longitudinal scan. The superior mesenteric vein lies over the inferior vena cava. The superior mesenteric vein dilates when obstructed by masses in the region of the pancreas.

FIGURE 5.19　(c)
Supine longitudinal scan. Tubular superior mesenteric vein is partially silhouetted by the enlarged pancreas in pancreatitis.

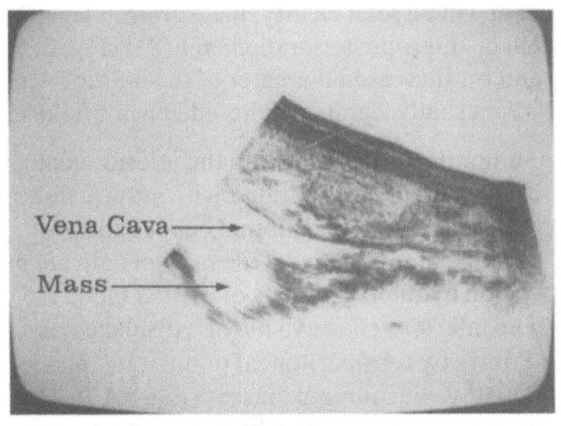

FIGURE 5-17

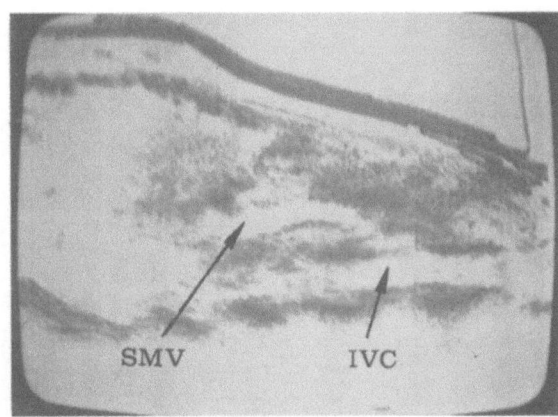

FIGURE 5-19 (a)

FIGURE 5-18

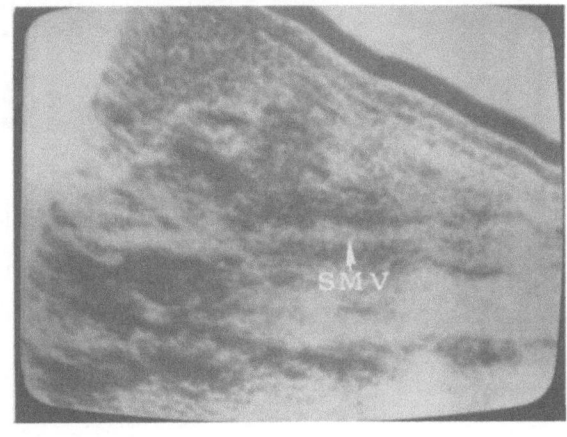

FIGURE 5-19 (b)

FIGURE 5-19 (c)

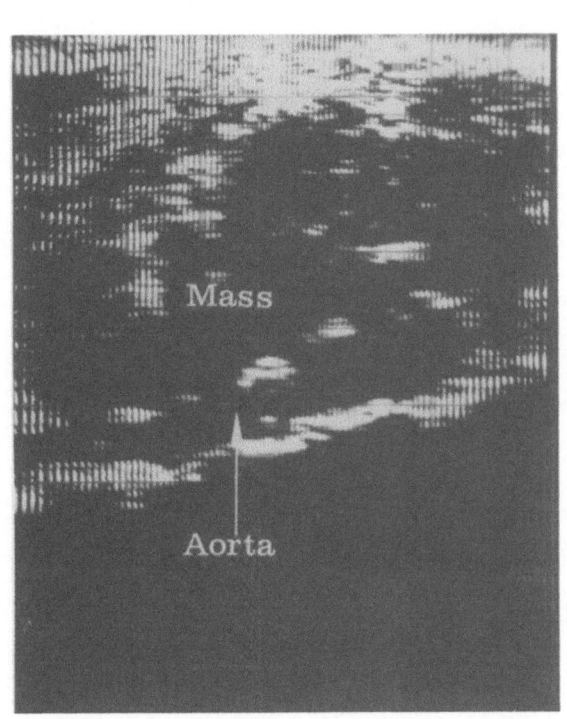

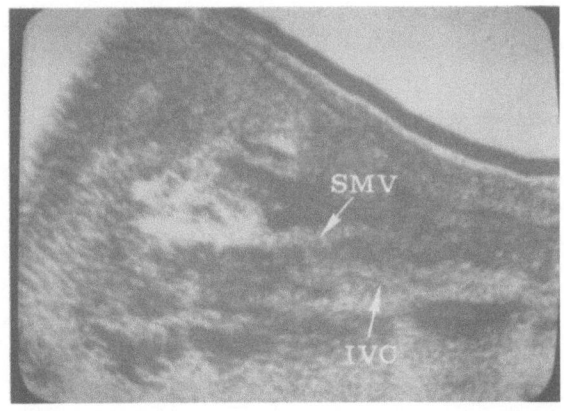

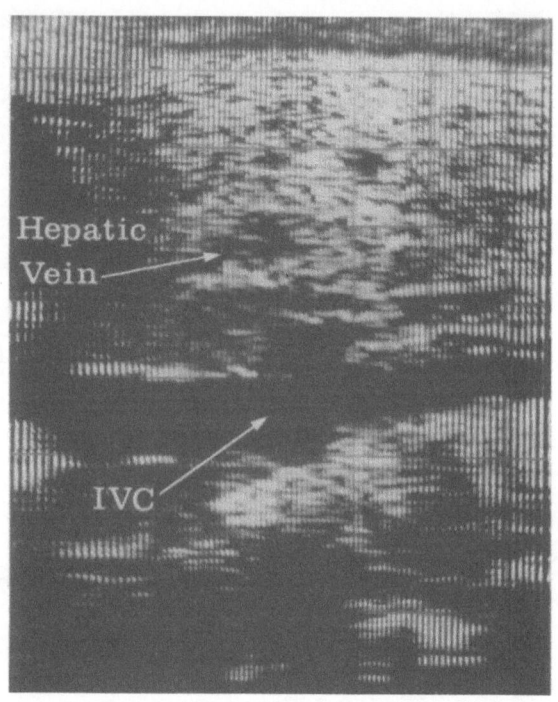

Hepatic Vein

IVC

FIGURE 5.20
Supine longitudinal scan. The inferior vena cava is distended due to cardiac failure. Part of the heart is well demonstrated above the liver parenchyma with the real-time scanner.

vein will be seen clearly, measuring at least 2 cm in anteroposterior diameter (83) (Fig. 5.16a and b). Increased diameter of the inferior vena cava usually signifies right-sided heart failure.

Tumor or thrombus within the inferior vena cava may be demonstrated with gray-scale or real-time scanners. Internal echoes and the absence of normal pulsatile motion indicate invasion by tumor or areas of clotted blood (27). The inferior vena cava may be displaced anteriorly by retroperitoneal tumors, lymphadenopathy, and adrenal masses (Fig. 5.17). The vena cava or aorta may be pushed posteriorly by pancreatic lesions (Fig. 5.18). Extrinsic obstruction by masses in or near the pancreas may cause the superior mesenteric vein to distend (Fig. 5.19a, b, and c). The venous system distends in pericardial effusion or right heart failure (Fig. 5.20). Study of the venous system may suggest a cardiac or hepatic etiology for hepatomegaly.

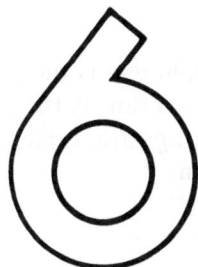

diaphragmatic sonography

GENERAL INTRODUCTION

The diaphragm separates the lungs from the abdomen and is affected in diseases of both cavities. Both diaphragmatic motion and contour may be demonstrated by ultrasound. Fluid collections above and below this muscular septum are easily identified. Since this is a simple procedure, it may be used as a screening test for diseases that affect motion of the diaphragm.

THE DIAPHRAGM

ANATOMY

The diaphragm is divided into a right and a left leaflet, which insert into an anteriorly located central tendon at the level of the xiphoid process. Between the right and left hemidiaphragms there are openings, from anterior to posterior, for the inferior vena cava, the esophagus, and the abdominal aorta, respectively.

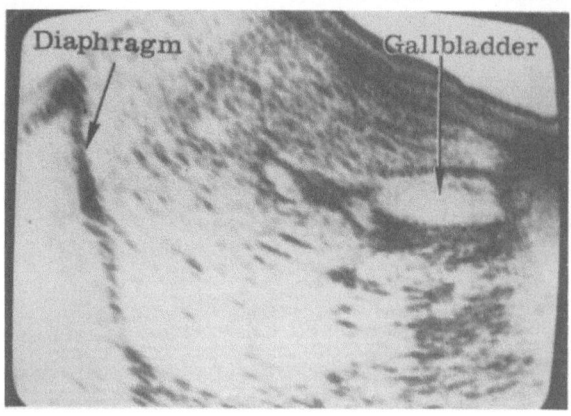

FIGURE 6-1

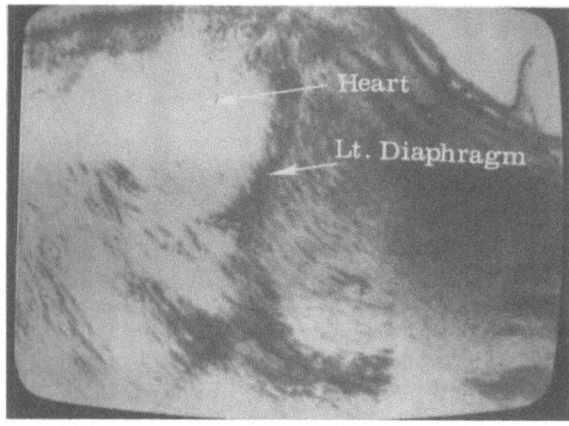

FIGURE 6-2

FIGURE 6-3

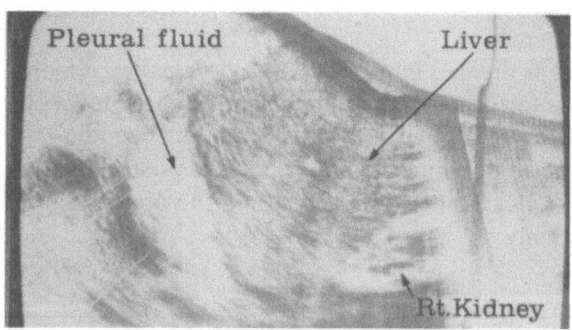

Superior to the right diaphragm is the right lung base; inferior is the dome of the right lobe of the liver.

Superior to the left diaphragm is the pericardium and left lung base, inferior, is the dome of the left lobe of the liver, gastric fundus, and upper pole of the spleen.

SONOANATOMY

The presence of the liver allows sound to reach the midsagittal plane of the right hemidiaphragm from the posterior aspect almost to the anterior attachment. The sonogram shows a smooth, mobile arc of dense echoes at the periphery of the liver (Fig. 6.1). Normally, the left hemidiaphragm cannot be imaged from anteriorly, and the portion that may be visualized by posterior scanning appears as a short, concave, echo-dense structure. Movement of the diaphragm depends both upon its own muscular contraction and the balance between respiratory excursions of the thoracic cage superiorly and intra-abdominal pressure exerted by the viscera on its under surface (Fig. 6.2).

SONOLAPAROTOMY

The right hemidiaphragm is easily imaged by arcing the transducer underneath the anterior

FIGURE 6.1
Supine longitudinal scan. The diaphragm on the right side is best imaged by sector scanning with the transducer angled under the rib cage. The outline is obtained during suspended respiration. Note the smooth arc-like configuration of the diaphragm. The left diaphragm is difficult to image in the normal patient.

FIGURE 6.2
Supine longitudinal scan. Longitudinal scan in the left paramedian plane demonstrates the left hemidiaphragm between the left lobe of the liver inferiorly and cardiac chamber superiorly.

FIGURE 6.3
Supine longitudinal scan. Echo-free zone above the right hemidiaphragm. Note the high through transmission phenomenon associated with the pleural fluid. One liter of pleural effusion was evacuated.

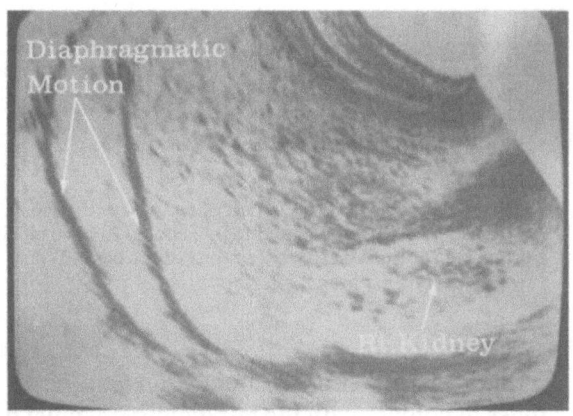

FIGURE 6-4

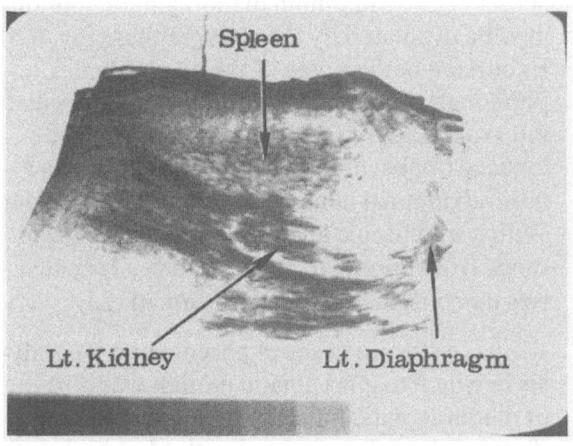

FIGURE 6-5 (a)

FIGURE 6-5 (b)

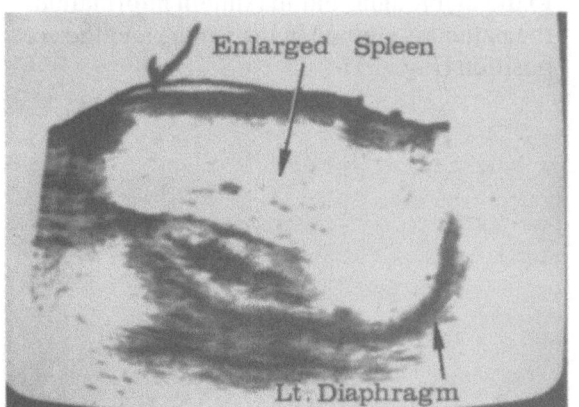

rib cage in the longitudinal plane. The extreme anterior aspect of the right hemidiaphragm may be appreciated by scanning with the patient prone. Similarly, the spleen permits evaluation of a posterior portion of the left hemidiaphragm. In the supine position, Trendelenburg's position with a fluid-filled stomach may increase visualization of the left hemidiaphragm (28). In the evaluation of subpulmonic effusion (Fig. 6.3), both supine and erect positions are used to estimate the amount of fluid and assess it as free or loculated. Diaphragmatic motion may be recorded on a single scan in expiration and inspiration (Fig. 6.4) or on an M-mode tracing with appropriate markers.

SONOPATHOLOGY

Supradiaphragmatic fluid appears as an echo-free area above the liver echoes of the diaphragm. This zone ceases at the pleural interface where another linear arc of echoes is noted (Fig. 6.3). The echo-free area, or free pleural fluid will decrease in size as the patient is moved from the erect to the recumbent position. Loculated fluid, or abscess, will not change in shape as the patient's position is altered.

A space-occupying mass in the left upper quadrant makes the left hemidiaphragm easy to image. Indeed, if the left diaphragm is visualized

FIGURE 6.4
Supine longitudinal scan. Proper evaluation of the diaphragmatic motion must be made in maximum inspiration and expiration. This measurement of respiratory excursion may be used as a baseline in the management of pulmonary diseases.

FIGURE 6.5 (a)
Supine longitudinal scan. The left diaphragm is clearly outlined. This occurs when the air-containing bowel is displaced by a good medium for sound transmission. It is common in splenomegaly, enlargement of the left lobe of the liver, and massive subdiaphragmatic fluid collections. Splenomegaly.

FIGURE 6.5 (b)
Supine longitudinal scan. The left diaphragm is well imaged. The gas containing organs in the left upper quadrant are displaced by the enlarged spleen of chronic leukemia.

CHAPTER 6: DIAPHRAGMATIC SONOGRAPHY

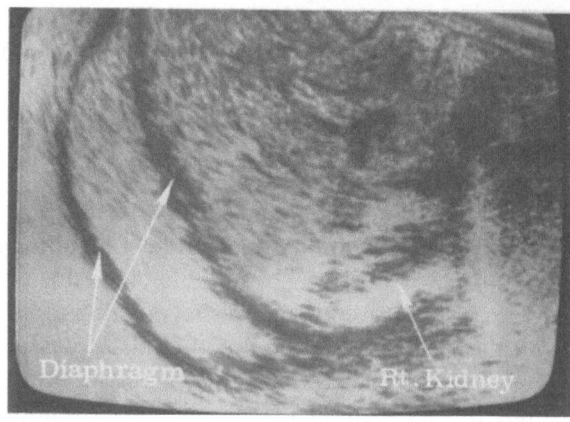

FIGURE 6-6

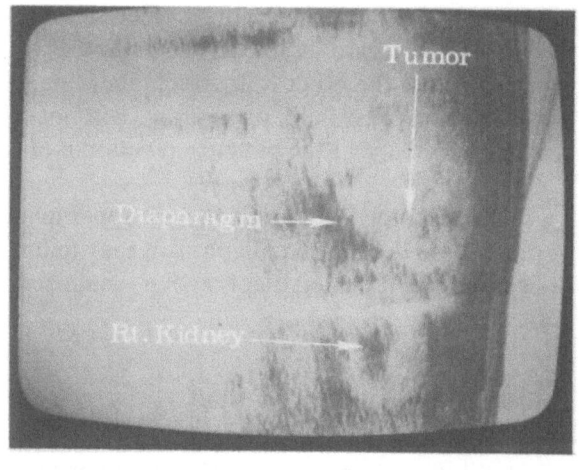

FIGURE 6-7

FIGURE 6.6
Supine longitudinal scan. Maximum excursion of the diaphragm. This is best evaluated with the transducer in a subcostal position. Several angulations are performed to obtain greatest movement.

FIGURE 6.7
Erect scan in right anterior axillary line. Above the renal outline the posterior hemidiaphragm is noted to have lost its normal curvature. Massive carcinoma of the base of the lung displacing diaphragm inferiorly.

without special effort, a sound-transmitting mass in contact with the left diaphragm must be suspected (Fig. 6.5). This has also been seen when sonic windows were created by marked hepatomegaly, ascites, and left subphrenic abscesses (28). Maximum diaphragmatic motion may be evaluated by the sonographer (Fig. 6.6). Excursion of the dome of the diaphragm in pulmonary disorders can be checked at regular intervals. Diaphragmatic motion may be decreased or absent in patients with ascites and intra-abdominal hemorrhage caused by trauma. With a subphrenic abscess, movement may range from normal to absent and in a recent series no consistent pattern was noted (28).

We have studied cases of phrenic nerve paralysis in which diaphragmatic motion was absent, of diaphragmatic flutter in hysterical patients (flutter is best documented with M-mode), and of eventration of the diaphragm presenting as a bulge in the normal arc of the diaphragm anteriorly. The diaphragm may be inverted or its normal excursion restricted by emphysema, subpulmonic effusion, and lung tumors adjacent to the diaphragm. Far maximum information, the patient is studied in the supine and the erect position (Fig. 6.7).

7 sonography of ascites

ASCITES

Intraperitoneal fluid assumes the form of either a transudate (low protein) or exudate (high protein). Common causes of transudates include portal obstruction, either intrahepatic or extrahepatic. Intrahepatic disease is usually cirrhosis of its many etiologies. Extrahepatic obstruction occurs with portal vein obstruction. Congestive heart failure, renal disease, and benign tumors of the ovary also cause ascites.

Exudates usually occur with inflammatory conditions of the peritoneum. The usual entities noted are infectious peritonitis and metastatic carcinoma, generally from the stomach, pancreas, and ovary. The peritoneum reacts to inflammation with a fibroblastic exudate that causes the peritoneum to adhere to other peritoneal surfaces, causing adhesions.

Ascites may be free or loculated. Free ascites is a transudate, except in the case of chylous ascites resulting from thoracic duct obstruction. Loculated ascites is seen with inflammatory conditions in which fluid is trapped in compart-

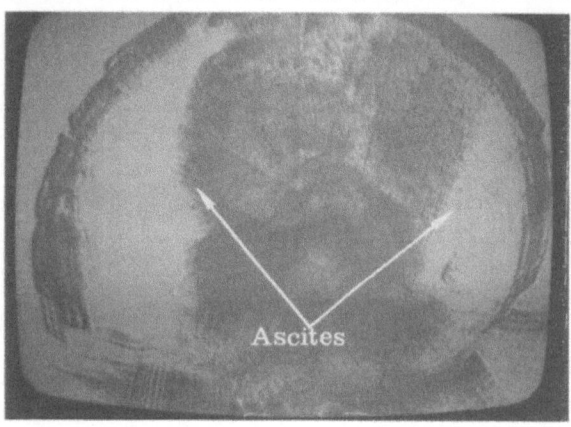

FIGURE 7.1

FIGURE 7.1
Supine transverse scan. Note atomic explosion configuration of massive ascites. The bowel and intra-abdominal organs are displaced medially. It is difficult to obtain information of diagnostic value. Rescanning when ascites is decreased is useful.

FIGURE 7.2
Supine longitudinal scan. Moderate amounts of ascites collect in the pelvis in the supine position. This echo-free fluid has the same echo pattern as the urine-filled bladder. Bowel loops projecting into the fluid are echogenic and produce a characteristic irregular outline to the ascitic fluid.

FIGURE 7.3
Supine longitudinal scan. Echo-free triangle of moderate amount of ascites. As fluid overflows the pelvic cavity it appears in the flank bordered by the abdominal wall, psoas muscle, and displaced bowel loops.

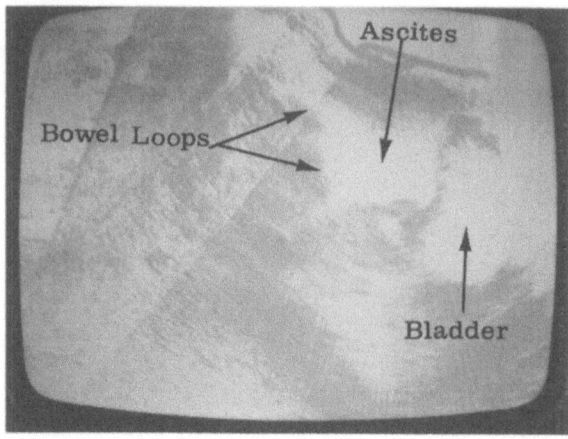

FIGURE 7.2

FIGURE 7.3

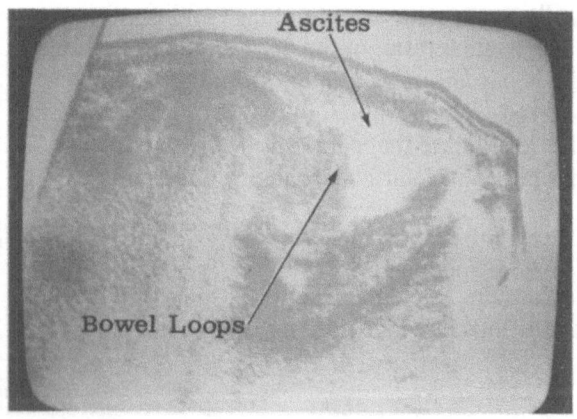

ments sealed by peritoneal adhesions. This may be localized to one area or diffusely situated throughout the intra-abdominal cavity (Fig. 7.1).

Minimal ascites may be detected with A-mode. As little as 100 ml of free fluid may be detected with the patient in the hand–knee position and the transducer placed under the anterior abdominal wall (21). Usually several minutes are allowed for the fluid to gravitate ventrally before the area is scanned.

Small amounts of ascites first collect in the pelvis by gravity. This collection appears as a sonolucent mass with angular borders anterosuperiorly due to indentation from overlying bowel (Fig. 7.2). Larger amounts overflow the pouch of Douglas and are directed by mesenteric reflections to specific regions (Fig. 7.3). These regions include the right paracolic gutter, the right lower quadrant at the lower end of the small bowel mesentery, and, with large amounts of fluid, the left lower quadrant along the superior border of the mesocolon (58). Ascites with tumor seedings or bacteria tends to loculate preferentially in these areas (Fig. 7.4).

Large amounts of fluid that extend up the paracolic gutters displace the bowel medially so that the scan resembles an atomic explosion (Fig. 7.1) and can distort the outline of the liver (Fig. 7.5). The air-containing intestine causes artifacts in supine scanning over the anterior abdomen. However, a moderate amount of ascitic

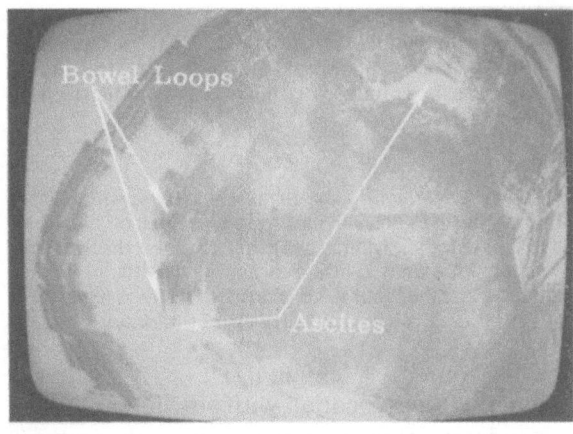

FIGURE 7.4

fluid provides an excellent scanning window when flank areas are scanned; large amounts of fluid prevent proper scanning. The lateral border of the medially displaced liver (Fig. 7.6a and b) and spleen can often be clearly delineated and elevation of the liver (Fig. 7.7), from the posteriorly located right kidney, may be demonstrated.

Although it is not possible to differentiate between benign and malignant ascites, transudates and exudates can be differentiated. Since transudates usually are free intraperitoneal fluid, they will change position with gravitational maneuvers. Exudates tend to loculate and will

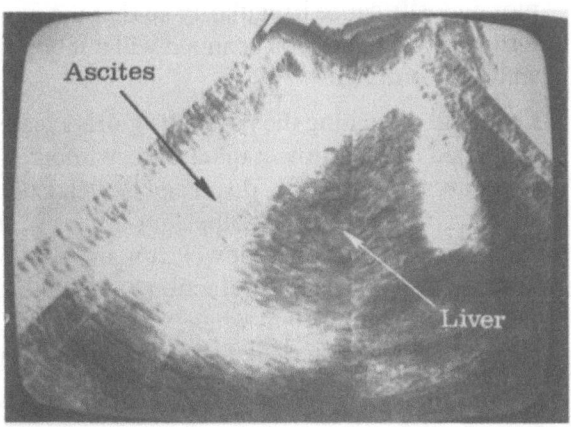

FIGURE 7.5

FIGURE 7.6 (a)

FIGURE 7.4
Supine transverse scan. Massive ascites usually prevents proper scanning. Loops of echogenic bowel project into the ascitic fluid. The bowel should float freely in the ascitic fluid and change with position. Fixation of bowel occurs in malignant and chronic inflammatory processes.

FIGURE 7.5
Supine longitudinal scan. The liver is shrunken and floats in an echo-free zone of ascites. Note elevation of the inferior liver edge from the retroperitoneal organs. Cirrhosis with ascites.

FIGURE 7.6 (a)
Supine transverse scan. Large amounts of ascitic fluid are situated in the paracolic gutters. Often a cirrhotic liver may be imaged by scanning through the right flank. Amorphous bowel artifacts are present anteriorly.

FIGURE 7.6 (b)
Supine longitudinal scan. A small attachment of echogenic parenchyma holds the liver to the retroperitoneal reflection. Diaphragm and anterior abdominal wall clearly outlined by ascitic fluid.

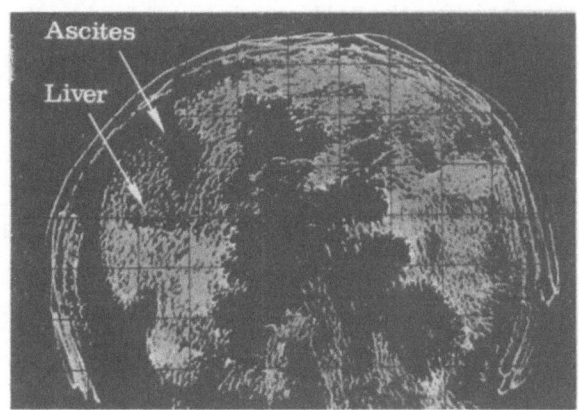

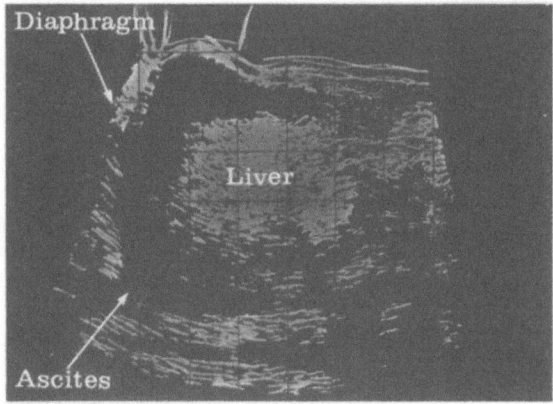

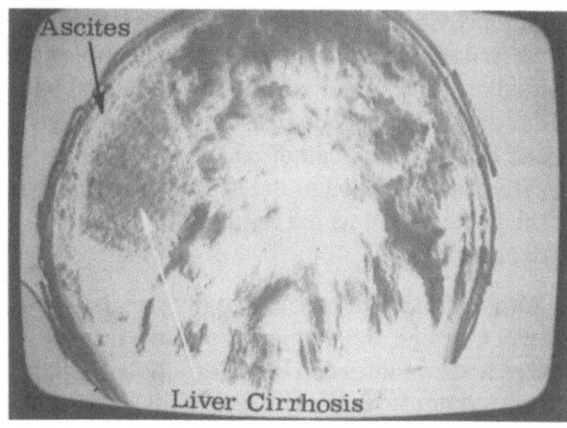

FIGURE 7.7

FIGURE 7.7
Supine longitudinal scan. Moderate ascites separating intra-abdominal organs from retroperitoneal structures. Anechoic fluid produces a sonolucent wedge between kidney and liver.

FIGURE 7.8
Supine longitudinal scan. In massive ascites without adhesions, the liver floats in the fluid and is lifted off the liver bed. Ascites with adhesions generally holds the liver adjacent to the kidney. The appearance of the "thumb-like" kidney and the "four finger shape" of the liver make the "mitten-sign" characteristic of cirrhotic ascites.

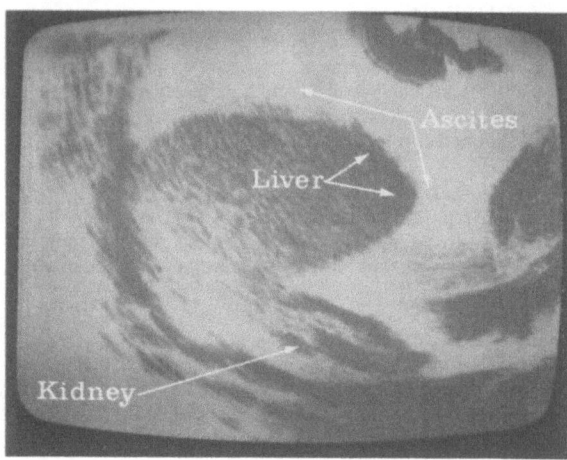

FIGURE 7.8

not alter their location with positioning. When exudates are in loculated cavities, the walls of the cavities will be seen as septations, which appear as linear echo patterns, in the echo-free fluid. Inflammatory changes in the walls or tumor deposits cause irregularity so that the posterior wall of the region scanned will not be smoothly outlined.

Free fluid ascending the paracolic gutters may be tapped over the lower quadrants, without perforating the medially displaced bowel. Loculated ascites implies that adhesions are preventing normal separation of bowel from the peritoneal surface. Ultrasonic detection of loculated ascites is very important when paracentesis is planned because the risk of bowel perforation is then increased.

Indeed, since the transducer may be easily placed over the pocket of trapped ascites, ultrasonically guided paracentesis is the method of choice when loculated fluid is present.

Excessive ascites prevents proper scanning of the abdomen; the examination should be repeated after the fluid is aspirated either blindly or through ultrasonic guided paracentesis.

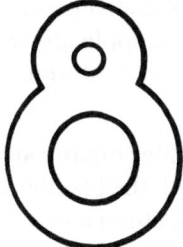

sonography in planning radiation therapy

GENERAL INTRODUCTION

B-scan echotomography is practical and accurate for demonstrating cross-sectional anatomy and displaying the morphology of organs altered by pathologic processes. Deep-seated tumors can be localized and tissue characteristics determined. Consequently, a plan for radiation therapy can be established by recording the patient's contour. Echotomographic information can be reliably and precisely incorporated into the treatment plan to decrease complications and increase the efficacy of the treatment. Sonography permits three-dimensional therapy analysis by the data displayed from right-angle sonograms. A strong echo appears at the surface of an organ or mass lesion because different tissues have different acoustic characteristics.

PATIENT CONTOUR

The patient contour can be obtained in any desired plane simply and accurately. At a very low gain setting, a single sweep of the transducer over the area of interest will give a contour tracing (6,7). Sonographic marking is more accurate than mechanical jigs, lead solder, plastic templates, or plaster. The transducer can be swept over a given region repeatedly. If the area of pathology is complex, multiple sections can be made for additional information.

Lung lesions, at the present time, cannot be evaluated by sonography because sound transmission through pulmonary tissue that contains air is absent. However, the thickness of the chest wall can be displayed so that treatment can be planned for carcinoma of the breast. This measurement is important because it is used to calculate beam energy and for tangential planning so that underlying lung tissue receives minimum irradiation (6).

LOCALIZATION OF DEEP LESIONS

Sonolaparotomy with different gain settings can be performed at the same time that the patient contour is scanned. Thus, the location and size of a space-occupying lesion relative to regional anatomy can be recorded. Echo-tomography to delineate deep-seated lesions and retroperitoneal lymphadenopathy is very useful. Enlarged lymph nodes in this area appear as sonolucent masses, with sharp margins anterior or anterolateral to the spine. This information may be obtained in both longitudinal and transverse scans. Echography is also valuable for staging carcinoma of the cervix, bladder, and prostate, since it detects enlarged lymph nodes in the pelvis and abdomen. For the same reason, sonography is important in assessing the extent of Hodgkin's disease and other lymphomas. Ascites, both free and loculated, can also be diagnosed.

ORGAN EVALUATION IN RADIATION THERAPY

Pelvic malignancy, especially in the uterus and cervix, can be outlined and tumor size and contour used to plan treatment. If intracavitary applicators are to be used, their position can be monitored by ultrasound. The echo from a radium-loaded tandem is quite strong. To calculate dosage, the position of the applicator with respect to the bladder as well as uterine width must be known.

Sonography detects bladder tumors and determines the degree to which the bladder wall is involved. Special transurethral and transrectal scanners are available, which may add more information for staging malignancies of the bladder and prostate.

Upper abdominal organs are also outlined and necrotic tumors demonstrated (31). The enlarged spleen in malignant disorders can be mapped three dimensionally and irradiated accordingly. The development of radiation fibrosis within irradiated organs is evidenced by the increased echogenicity of the organ parenchyma (77). The kidneys can be localized and their size and position determined so that they can be shielded appropriately during treatment (64).

DELINEATION OF PORT MARGINS

The portal of treatment can be outlined over the abdomen, retroperitoneum, or pelvis. Breaking the contact between transducer and skin surface produces a mark on the scan. Thus, the periphery of a specific region can be marked on the scan and the skin painted with indelible ink. In every step of marking, the transducer should be elevated slightly from the skin surface; the margin is obtained by visual display. A polaroid picture is taken as a baseline and compared with polaroid pictures of future examinations. In this manner port margins can be decreased as needed.

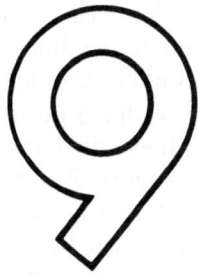

retroperitoneal sonography

GENERAL INTRODUCTION

It is difficult to evaluate the retroperitoneal area by ordinary radiographic methods, since space-occupying lesions must be far-advanced in this region before they can be detected. And, despite the standard roentgenographic work-up for patients, which includes intravenous urography, barium enema, lymphangiography, retroperitoneal air insufflation, and angiography, the nature of the lesion may remain unclear. This is especially true of avascular masses and surgery may be required for definitive diagnosis. However, sonolaparotomy, as a noninvasive, safe, and simple technique for detecting, evaluating, and differentiating retroperitoneal lesions, has been rewarding.

THE RETROPERITONEUM

ANATOMY

The retroperitoneum is best appreciated when it is divided into upper and lower retroperitoneal spaces at the level of the posterior iliac crest. The upper retroperitoneal space is subdivided into anterior and posterior compartments. From right to left, the anterior division contains the ascending colon, descending duodenum, pancreas, and descending colon. The posterior division contains the right renal fascia, fat and right kidney, upper portion of the left psoas muscle, left kidney, and left renal fat and fascia. The lower retroperitoneal space contains the ascending colon, body of the right psoas muscle, right ureter, aortic bifurcation or right and left iliac artery and vein, body of the left psoas muscle, and descending colon. Major lymph node chains follow the iliac vessels.

SONOANATOMY

Sonographically, the retroperitoneal space is divided into upper and lower sections at the plane of the umbilicus or iliac crest (54). The sonographer should identify as many structures as possible in the supine, prone, or lateral projections. The bony pelvis prevents visualization of the lower compartment from posterior projections. Details of the sonoanatomy of each retroperitoneal organ are described separately.

SONOLAPAROTOMY

Both supine and prone positions are used when the upper retroperitoneum is scanned. Prone is ideal for studying the kidneys and upper psoas muscles. The supine position must be used for structures that lie anterior to the spine, since the sonic shadow of the vertebral column prevents this approach. In the normal patient the most prominent structure is the iliopsoas muscle. Transverse sonolaparotomy from the level of the iliac crest towards the feet demonstrates the psoas portion of the muscle as an ovoid, sonolucent band adjacent to the vertebral column The lack of central echoes, characteristic of the renal collecting system, within the psoas muscle prevents mistaking this structure for the kidney. In longitudinal scanning, the psoas muscles appear as bilaterally symmetric sonolucent

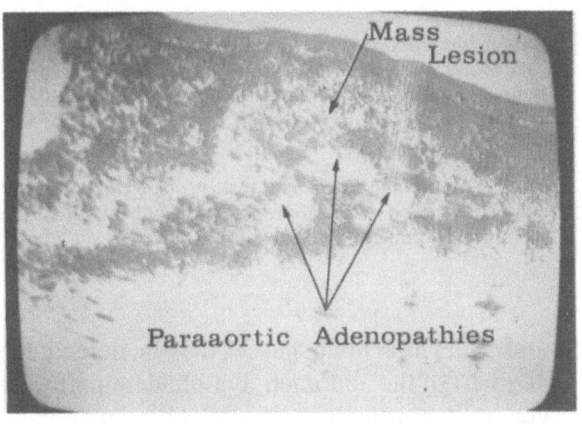

FIGURE 9.1 (a)

regions, usually best visualized between 5 and 7 cm from the midline.

The lower retroperitoneum can only be examined with commercial scanners when the patient is in the supine position or transrectally with special endoscanners. It is best to have the bladder full to provide a cystic anatomic reference point.

SONOPATHOLOGY

In the upper abdomen enlarged lymph nodes are usually seen as rounded masses in close proximity to the abdominal aorta (Fig. 9.1a, b,

FIGURE 9.1 (a)
Supine longitudinal scan. Discrete clusters of anechoic and echogenic masses obscure the normal aortic outline. Hodgkin's disease.

FIGURE 9.1 (b)
Supine transverse scan. Periaortic lymphadenopathy presenting as multiple anechoic masses. Left para-aortic lymph nodes displace the left kidney laterally.

FIGURE 9.1 (c)
Supine transverse scan. Multiple anechoic masses in the periaortic region. The real-time scanner may detect the pulsatile aorta and the inferior vena cava.

FIGURE 9.1 (b)

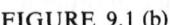

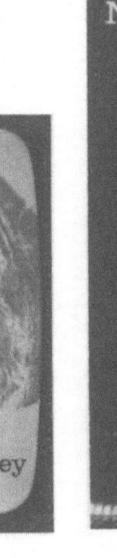

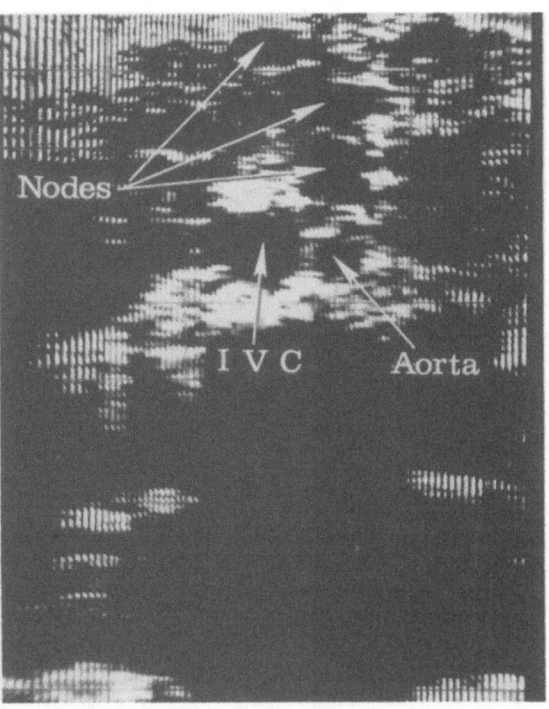

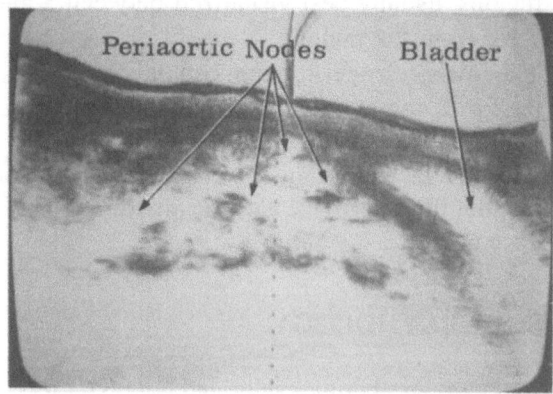

FIGURE 9.2 (a)

FIGURE 9.2 (b)

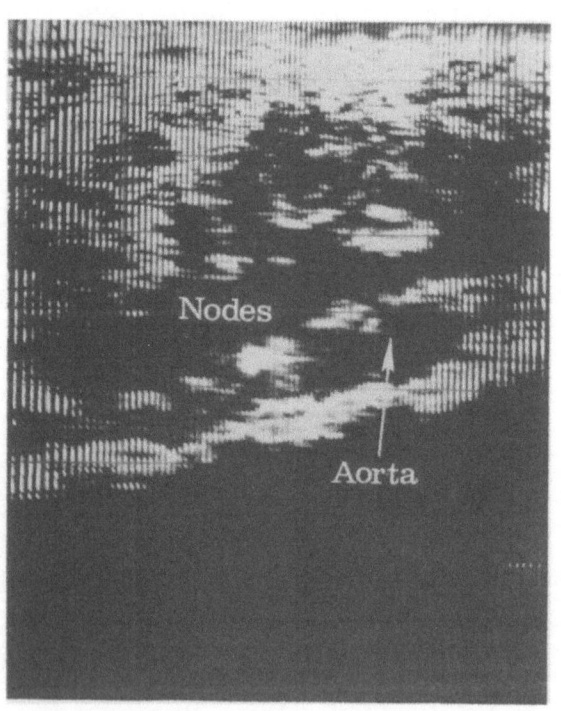

FIGURE 9.2 (a)
Supine longitudinal scan. Midline scan over the aorta fails to reveal the normal aortic outline. Masses of enlarged lymph nodes adjacent to the aorta silhouette the aortic walls and obscure its normal borders.

FIGURE 9.2 (b)
Supine longitudinal scan. The aorta is displaced dorsally by echo-free matted lymph nodes. Note the concave shape of the normally straight anterior aortic wall.

and c). Lymph node masses may be detected in any part of the abdomen; lymphadenopathy generally appears sonolucent. These masses may retain an echo-free pattern even at high-gain settings (Fig. 9.2a and b) because the diseased lymph nodes are acoustically homogeneous.

During the scan, every attempt is made to image the spine in order to establish a boundary distal to the lesion. A lymph node mass adjacent to the wall of the aorta makes it difficult to verify the position of this vessel within the tumor mass (Fig. 9.1c). The echo silhouette sign of lymphadenopathy adjacent to the aorta, actually obliterating the anterior aortic wall, has been noted with B-scan, gray scale, and real-time scanner. Indeed, such a cluster of periaortic lymph nodes may mimic an aortic aneurysm. Generally these nodal aggregates have an irregular, lobulated outline as compared to an abdominal aortic aneurysm. Scanning other areas of the abdomen or retroperitoneum may demonstrate other sonolucent lesions distinct from the abdominal aorta. The presence of other foci of lymphadenopathy rules against the possibility of an aortic aneurysm. We have noted lymphadenopathy appearing as discrete masses, sonolucent layers covering the aorta, and multiple tumors that may elevate the aorta and inferior vena cava anteriorly (Fig. 9.3).

Retroperitoneal tumors may be demonstrated either by prone or supine echotomography. These masses may displace the kidneys and intra-abdominal organs by spread into the mesentery (Fig. 9.2). Tumors with internal degeneration may be observed to have multiple internal echoes with a high through transmission phenomenon.

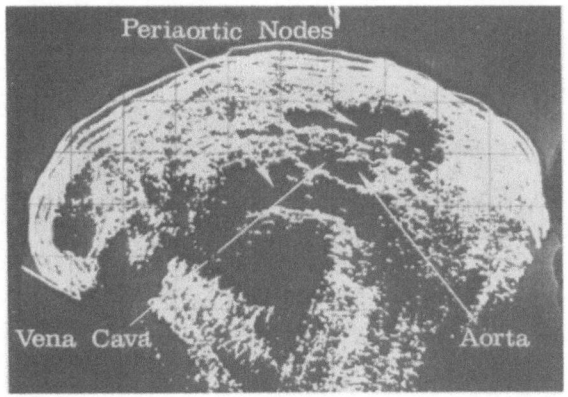

FIGURE 9.3

FIGURE 9.3
Supine transverse scan. The aorta and inferior vena cava are elevated from the spine by sheets of lymph nodes. These masses are echo free at high sensitivity.

FIGURE 9.4
Right decubitus scan. The right kidney is displaced anteriorly. An ovoid echo-free zone replaces the paravertebral musculature. Cold abscess in patient with tuberculosis.

FIGURE 9.5
Prone longitudinal scan. Echo-free retroperitoneal hematoma pushes the lower pole of the kidney anteriorly. Leaking aortic aneurysm.

Retroperitoneal fluid collections may be noted by an echo-free zone. It may be impossible to differentiate between hemorrhage, abscess (Fig. 9.4), and sterile fluid (54). If the patient is symptomatic, study of the aorta is indicated to rule out a leaking aortic aneurysm as a cause of retroperitoneal blood (Fig. 9.5).

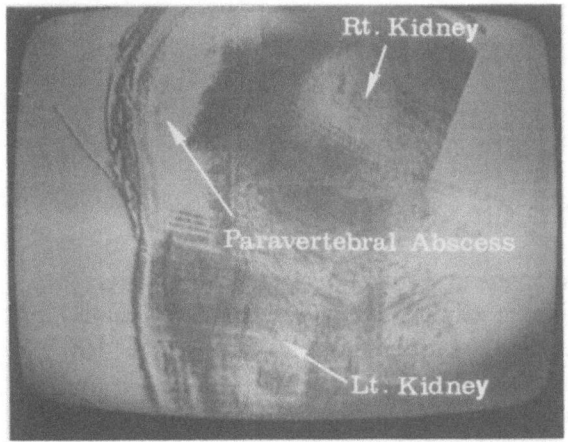

FIGURE 9.4

FIGURE 9.5

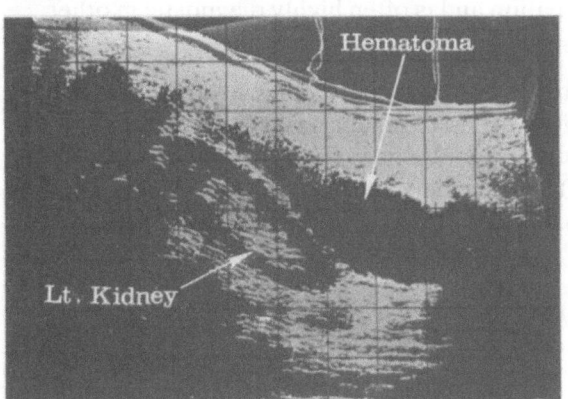

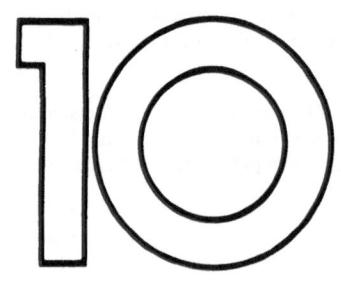

renal
sonography

by Robert Bard, M.D.

GENERAL INTRODUCTION

Thorough diagnostic investigations and a general increased life span has increased the incidence with which renal masses are detected by intravenous urograms. The high accuracy of ultrasound in the diagnosis of renal cysts has made sonography the test of choice and spurred investigation of a multitude of pathologic processes of the kidneys and pararenal organs by ultrasound. Of the various modalities, ultrasonography is the technique that yields considerable diagnostic information with the least risk, expense, or trauma to the patient. Often, ultrasonic investigation is the only practical method for diagnosing renal masses in the geriatric population and is often highly diagnostic in other medical and surgical renal disorders.

Following intravenous urography, sonic evaluation is the next step in the workup of renal masses. Ultrasonically guided renal cyst puncture has achieved great diagnostic accuracy (39) and is widely used in clinical practice. The following is a list of applications of ultrasound in renal disease.

1. Normal kidney
2. Simple cyst, multiple cysts

3. Localization for cyst puncture, aspiration, and renal biopsy
4. Solid masses with or without internal degeneration
5. Renal transplant pathology
6. Multicystic and polycystic kidney disease
7. Hydronephrosis
8. Renal calculus
9. Adrenal tumors and perirenal lesions
10. Renal aplasia, renal ectopia, horseshoe kidney, ptotic and displaced kidney

ANATOMY

The paired kidneys, with their characteristic shape, are located retroperitoneally in the lumbar region. Their outer contour is smooth, laterally, with a convex border, whereas the concave medial aspect has a central invagination for renal vessels and for the origin of the renal pelvis. This area is called the hilus of the kidney. The left kidney is usually 1 or 2 cm cephalad to the right and tends to be the larger of the two varying in size from 8 to 13 cm in length. The kidneys move with respiratory motion; however, this is not significant during normal quiet respiration.

The close relationship of the kidney to the posteriorly located back muscles produces the observed lateral displacement. The psoas major muscle is smaller cranially than caudally; hence the greater lateral deviation of the lower pole of the kidney accounts for the usual oblique plane of this organ. In the lateral decubitus position the kidney nearest the transducer undergoes a medical and anterior shift.

THE KIDNEY

SONOANATOMY

The normal kidney has an ovoid configuration in the transverse plane and is elliptical in the longitudinal axis. In the normal kidney, both

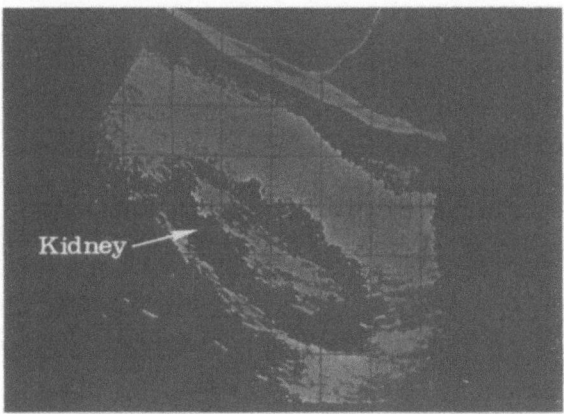

FIGURE 10.1
Prone longitudinal scan. Distal to the retroperitoneal musculature is the elliptical sonolucent outline of the renal cortex with the echogenic central calyceal echoes. B-mode at medium sensitivity.

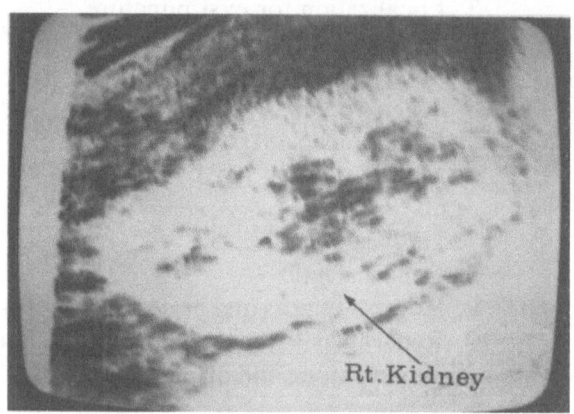

FIGURE 10.2 (a)

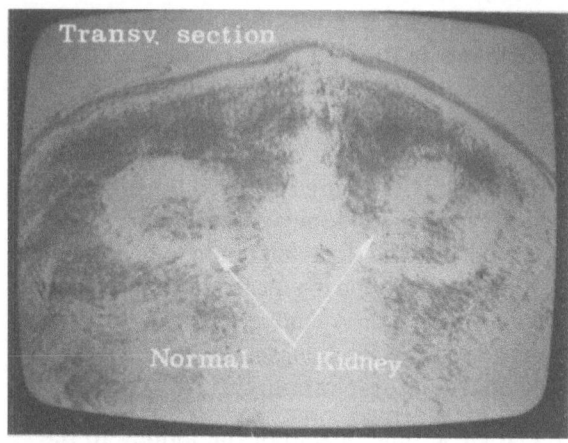

FIGURE 10.2 (b)

FIGURE 10.2 (c)

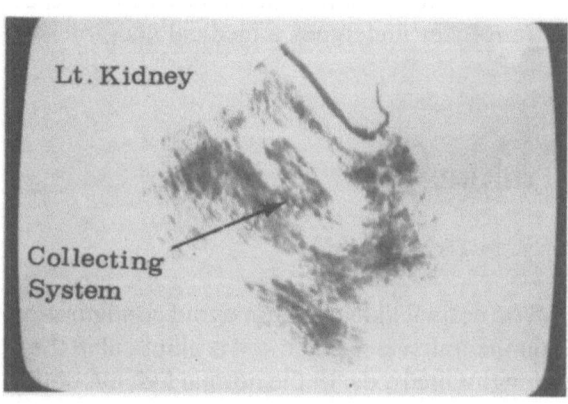

sonolucent (black) and sonopaque (white) echo patterns can be produced. At low sensitivity, the cortex of the kidney is sonolucent and the pelvicalyceal system appears as a speckled echo pattern extending medially from the center of each kidney. This central echo pattern represents calyces and vascular structures within the renal sinus (37) (Fig. 10.1). At a higher sensitivity setting, the renal parenchyma fills-in with echoes. During routine scanning, the pelvicalyceal system appears as a sonopaque configuration following the sonolucent oblique course of the renal cortex (80).

Improved resolution with gray-scale systems may show a scalloped outer border of the central calyceal echoes. The renal parenchyma appears echo free (colorless or light gray), and calyceal echoes are dark gray (Fig. 10.2a and b). The region of the renal sinus appears when the pelvicalyceal echoes extend to the ventral and medial border of the kidney (Fig. 10.2c).

The kidney has a characteristic appearance on the A-scope, with high-amplitude echoes, corresponding to the anterior and posterior wall, and several low-amplitude central echoes from the collecting system (Fig. 10.3). The image of the kidney with the real-time scanner is similar to the conventional B-scan (Fig. 10.4a and b).

Anterior to the right kidney (medial to lateral) lie the duodenal sweep and hepatic flexure. Anterior to the left kidney is the tail of the pancreas and the splenic flexure. The aorta is medial to the left kidney, and the left renal vein

FIGURE 10.2   (a)
Prone longitudinal scan. Note the scalloped outer border of the renal collecting system echoes. This is a normal variation noted with the high resolution of gray scale.

FIGURE 10.2   (b)
Prone transverse scan. Ovoid echo-poor renal outlines appear on either side of the sonic shadow of the spine. Within each kidney are the central dark echoes of the collecting system.

FIGURE 10.2   (c)
Prone longitudinal scan. The homogeneous echo pattern of the collecting system extends anteriorly. This region is called the renal sinus and contains the renal pelvis and renal vessels.

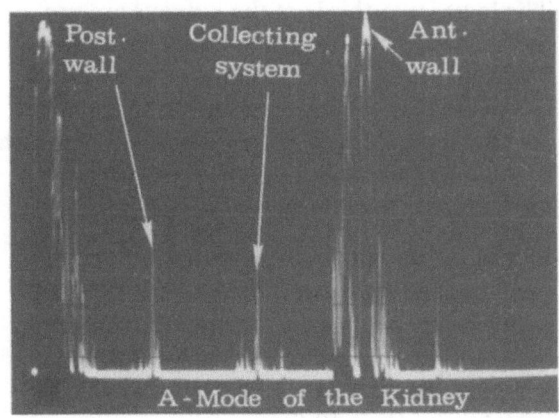

FIGURE 10.3

crosses anterior to the aorta (Fig. 10.5). The adrenal glands generally lie superomedially to the upper pole of each kidney. The posterior edge of the liver is separated from the right kidney by perirenal fat and fascia. Occasionally, the spleen may be located above the left kidney (Fig. 10.6) and in this position it may be difficult to separate this organ from the upper pole of the kidney. Careful scanning technique is important to prevent misdiagnosing a normal spleen as a renal mass lesion. The lateral decubitus position is often helpful in separating the spleen from the left kidney (Fig. 10.7).

FIGURE 10.3
A-mode of the kidney. Characteristic high-amplitude proximal and distal wall echoes with scattered low-amplitude echoes corresponding to the pelvicalyceal system. This distance between kidney and the skin may be measured from the calibrated oscilloscope.

FIGURE 10.4 (a)
Prone longitudinal scan. The renal cortex, perirenal fat, and perinephric musculature shown at medium sensitivity with the real-time scanner as echo-free zones. Echogenic collecting system.

FIGURE 10.4 (b)
Prone longitudinal scan. At high sensitivity, the renal parenchyma remains echo poor while the perirenal fat and muscles fill in with echoes.

FIGURE 10.4 (a)

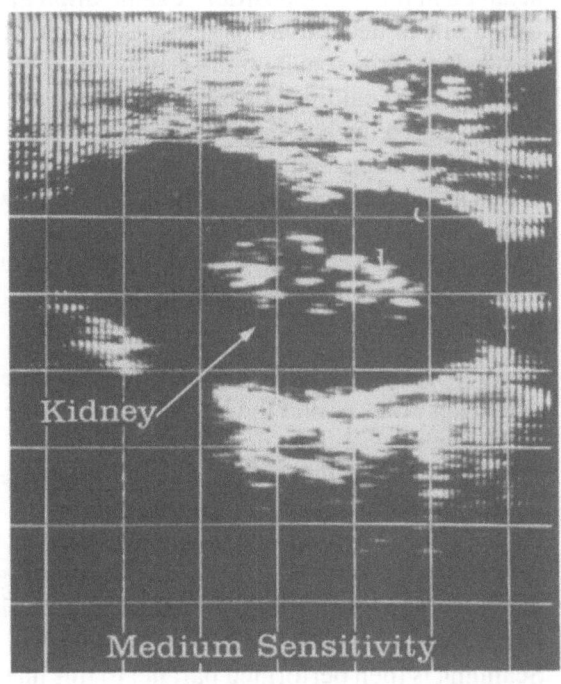

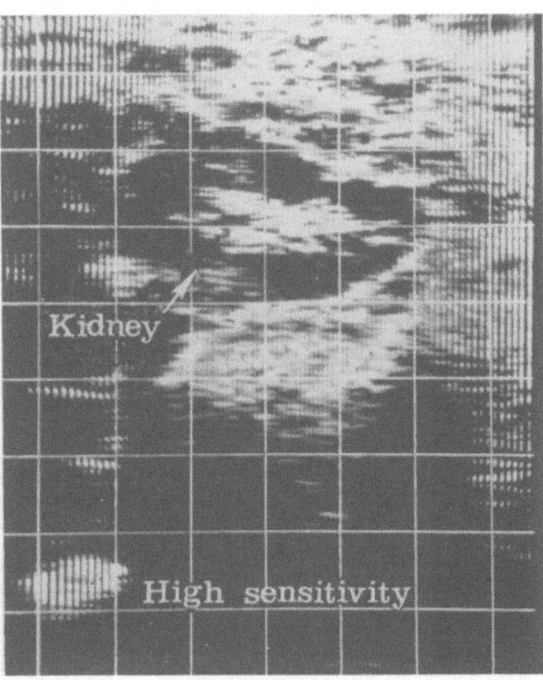

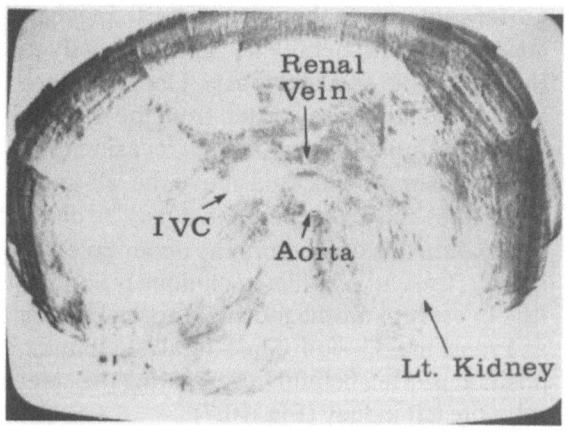

FIGURE 10.5
Supine transverse scan. The anechoic tubular left renal vein crosses over the aorta as it joins the inferior vena cava.

FIGURE 10.6
Prone longitudinal scan. The sonolucent spleen often lies adjacent to the upper pole of the left kidney. This may be confused with a renal cyst if high sensitivity is not used. Sector scanning serves to more clearly demonstrate the splenorenal demarcation.

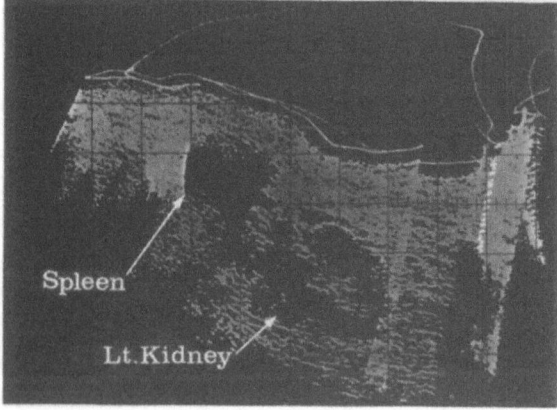

The lower two-thirds of the kidneys are protected posteriorly (medial to lateral) by the psoas muscle, quadratus lumborum, and aponeurosis of the transverse abdominus muscle. The posterior aspect of the diaphragm, the 12th rib on the right, and the 11th and 12th ribs on the left cross the upper third of the kidneys.

During ultrasonic investigation, the sonographer must be aware of the confusing rib shadows produced as the sound beam is blocked by bony structures, and wedge-shaped echo patterns are generated by lung tissue in each intercostal space (Fig. 10.8).

SONOLAPAROTOMY

A combination of B-scan with simultaneous A-mode display is used to investigate renal masses. B-scan, gray-scale, or real-time display localizes the mass three dimensionally. The presence or absence of echoes distinguishes solid from cystic space-occupying lesions and is best demonstrated with A-mode.

Sonography follows physical examination and intravenous urography. The patient is initially scanned in the prone position; examination in the supine or decubitus position may be added as needed. If the renal outline is not well defined in the unmodified prone position, the degree to which the body is extended can be reduced by placing a pillow under the abdomen. If this maneuver does not produce satisfactory visualization, hyperextension may improve imaging. Interruption of respiration aids resolution in B-scanning and is essential for greater detail with gray scale.

The general renal area is searched for the upper and lower poles to find the best scanning plane for the kidneys and the proper angulation for the transducer. When the upper and lower poles have been outlined, and appropriate marks made on the skin to localize the poles on the surface of the body, lines are drawn connecting the upper and lower poles of each kidney. Each line represents the long axis of the kidney. Scanning is then performed parallel to this line

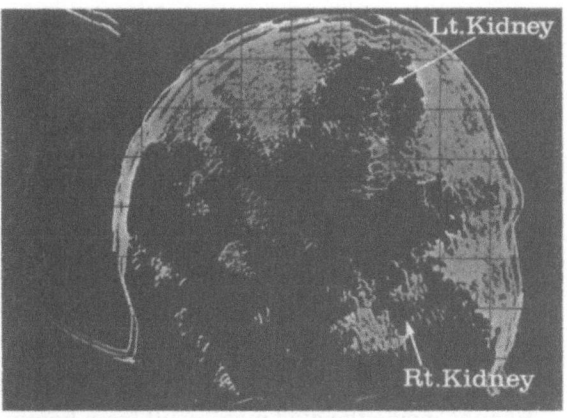

FIGURE 10.7
Left lateral decubitus scan. The area of interest is adjacent to the transducer. The left renal outline is more clearly imaged than the right. Note that the left kidney moves anterior and medial in this position, which is ideal for separating the spleen from the kidney.

FIGURE 10.8
Prone longitudinal scan. The calyceal echo pattern is divided and the distal renal wall is lost due to the sonic shadow effect of the rib.

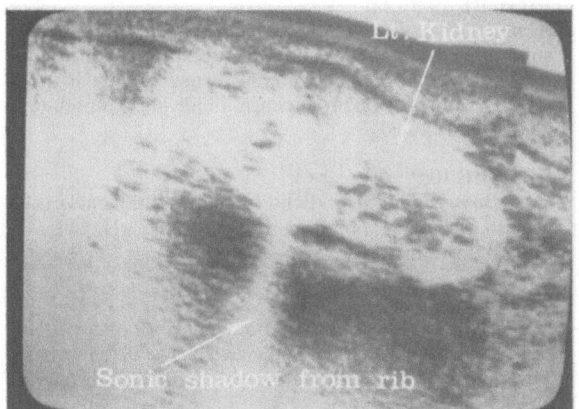

in the longitudinal position until the entire renal parenchyma is visualized. The kidney lies at an angle, with respect to the skin of the back. This angle, which varies for each kidney, depends upon retroperitoneal musculature and local pathologic changes. Longitudinal scanning will show the position of the kidney in this plane. In transverse scanning the angle of the transducer is adjusted so that the sound beam strikes the kidney perpendicular to the plane of the renal outline. A 2.25-MHz transducer gives sufficient detail for routine imaging. Generally, scans are made at 1-cm intervals and are continued until both kidneys are well-demonstrated from the upper to the lower poles.

If a solid mass is identified, supine scanning is performed since it is important to evaluate the mass from the anterior aspect. Also, the sonic shadow of the vertebrae may obscure enlarged para-aortic lymph nodes. Using the supine or erect position will aid in diagnosing the ptotic kidney.

Abdominal x-ray films and intravenous urograms can guide the sonographer to the renal location and area of pathology. At low sensitivity, the mass outlined may be compared with the size of the mass on the x-ray film; the nature of the lesion is ascertained by increasing the sensitivity. Change of sensitivity is usually unnecessary with gray-scale display.

SONOPATHOLOGY

RENAL CYST

The following criteria are used to diagnose a renal cyst:

1. Echo-free zone within the mass due to a homogeneous medium.
2. Sharp definition of the distal wall of the mass and a smooth contour to this surface, due to the large change in acoustic impedance at the cyst wall interface and the parabolic shape reflecting more sound back to the transducer.
3. Greater energy of the sound beam due to minimal attenuation of sound tra-

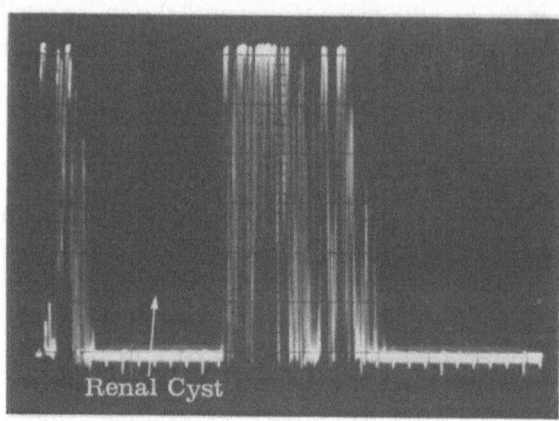

FIGURE 10.9 (a)

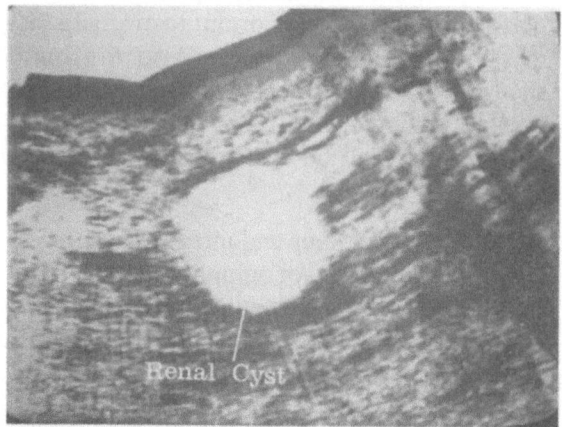

FIGURE 10.9 (b)

FIGURE 10.9 (c)

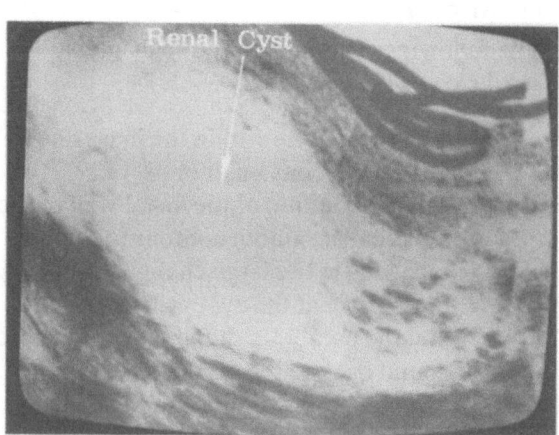

versing the homogeneous fluid-fllilled medium, resulting in increased through transmission and therefore increased echo density distal to the lesion. This effect is more pronounced with a larger cystic mass (Fig. 10.9a through d).

The precise gain setting that fills-in a cyst with artifactual echoes is a matter of experience with a specific instrument. A suspected cyst should be compared with a known cystic mass standard, such as the bladder.

Echoes inside the cyst may result from hemorrhage, septations, tumor, infection, or respiratory motion. One or two strong echoes usually indicates a septum within a cyst (48). Diagnostic accuracy using A-mode alone was 95 percent in one series (25). Renal cysts in the older age groups are commonly multiple (26) (Fig. 10.10).

Percutaneous cyst puncture
Ultrasonically guided cyst puncture is most often used to diagnose renal cysts. The cystic lesion may be localized with the B-scan and echoes from the puncture needle detected as the needle is inserted into the skin. The transducer must be at right angles to the needle for optimum visualization. This approach is easier with the real-time scanner.

We prefer the puncture transducer for greater accuracy. The patient is scanned for optimal localization of the cyst. In combination with the B-scan, we use the calibrated A-scope to find

FIGURE 10.9　(a)
A-mode of renal cyst at high sensitivity. The flat baseline superimposed upon the calibrated oscilloscope represents the size of the cyst in the scanning plane. Note the high through transmission producing multiple high amplitude distal wall echoes.

FIGURE 10.9　(b)
Prone longitudinal scan. Echo-free lower pole renal cyst with sharp demarcation from renal substance. Head is toward the right.

FIGURE 10.9　(c)
Prone longitudinal scan. Anechoic renal cyst distorts the calyceal echo pattern of the upper pole. The distal wall is better outlined than the anterior wall. Note high through transmission.

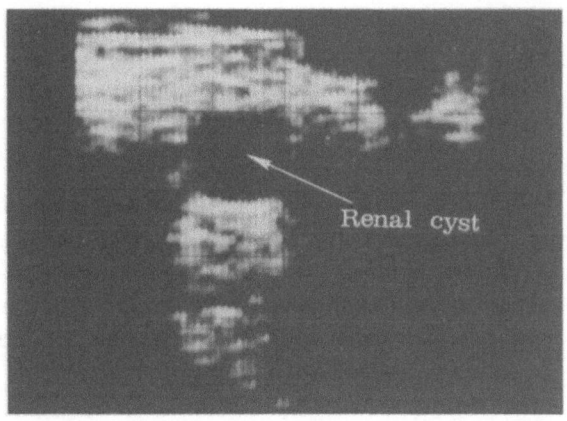

FIGURE 10.9 (d)

FIGURE 10.9   (d)
Prone transverse scan. Renal cyst with real-time scanner. Sharp concave distal wall with high through transmission. Absence of internal echoes.

FIGURE 10.10
Prone longitudinal scan. Two anechoic areas are visualized in one slice. The outline of the kidney is severely distorted. Multiple renal cysts are common in elderly patients. The opposite kidney should be studied for cystic changes.

the depth of the cyst from the surface and to measure proximal and distal walls. The distance from the skin to the middle of the cyst is determined and marked on the needle. Then the length of the special puncture transducer, through which the needle must pass, is added. The needle is advanced into the cyst while the A-scope is monitored constantly. When the needle enters the cyst, a "needle echo" is often imaged between the echoes from the cyst walls. Visualization of proximal and distal cyst walls with respect to the needle may also be recorded by M-mode and the position of the needle is adjusted accordingly. The needle is placed in the center of the cyst so that sufficient fluid may be aspirated without decompressing the distal wall, which may obstruct the orifice of the needle.

After the cyst is aspirated an air contrast study is usually performed to visualize the inner walls of the lesion. The volume of fluid in the echo-free area can be estimated, since cystic lesions usually approximate the volume of a sphere. Using the diameter of the lesion in question, its volume may be obtained from a standard nomogram. Optimally, half of the fluid is removed. One-half of the volume evacuated is reinjected as radiopaque contrast and the remaining one-half as air. This completely reconstitutes the original volume of the lesion and gives excellent contrast-coating to its walls. The outline of the lesion is compared with that of the contrast-filled region. If the contrast-outlined structure is smaller than the original lesion or irregular, a necrotic tumor or malignancy of the wall of the cyst must be suspected. Care must be taken to completely reexpand the cyst, otherwise the partially collapsed walls may simulate an internal filling defect. When a small cystic mass is

FIGURE 10.10

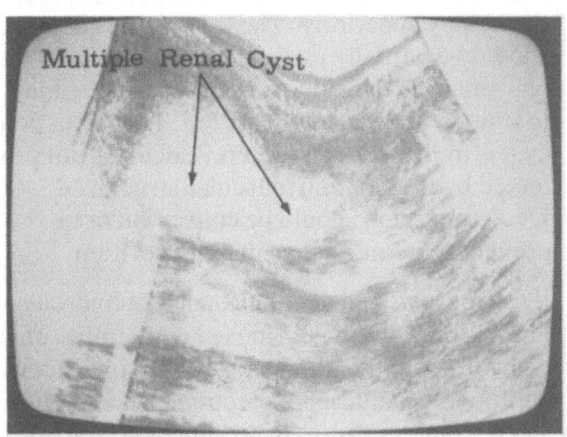

aspirated, only sufficient fluid for diagnostic purposes is removed to prevent the cyst wall from collapsing. If the cyst completely collapses, attempts to replace the contents with air and contrast may fail.

After the cyst has been punctured, the patient is sent to the x-ray department for AP, PA, erect, Trendelenburg position, and right and left lateral decubitus view films so that all regions of the cyst wall are visualized. Follow-up films should be taken at 24- and 48-hour intervals to evaluate the effect of decompression of the cyst. If no contrast is demonstrated on the 24-hour film, it is concluded that the contents of the cyst has leaked out continuously. Certain contrast has been used to cause sclerosis of cysts, but the febrile reactions are undesirable. Approximately 50 percent of aspirated cysts or of cysts instilled with contrast will recur at a later date (42). The aspirate is submitted for cytologic study and analyzed for fat and LDH (lactic dehydrogenase). Tumors and infected cysts contain high fat and LDH levels; benign cysts are low in both. It is felt that the potential for tumor spread into adjacent tissue by percutaneous puncture techniques is not great (81).

Therapeutic Indications for Ultrasonically Guided Puncture

Peripelvic cysts may cause hydronephrosis by obstructing the renal pelvis or proximal ureter. Decompression is indicated to relieve obstruction. The vector force of a large cyst of the upper pole pushes the kidney inferiorly while the effect of a large cyst of the lower pole displaces the kidney superiorly. These two types of cysts should be partially evacuated to prevent displacement of the kidney, which is more subject to trauma in the caudal position. The lower pole cyst is more prone to rupture, since it is not protected by the ribs and muscular structures. Decompression should be conservative to prevent extreme change in renal position.

Pyonephrosis and decompression of hydronephrosis may also be diagnosed under ultrasonic control. After the ultrasonic diagnosis of hydronephrosis is confirmed, percutaneous puncture and decompression may be indicated. We prefer to place the needle through the lateral, inferior aspect of the kidney to avoid injury to major renal vessels. A guide wire and drainage catheter are inserted into the renal pelvis. After the guide wire is withdrawn, urine or pus may be drained through the catheter. After the contents are decompressed, antegrade pyelography may be performed by injecting radiopaque contrast into the pelvicalyceal system and allowing the ureters to be filled by gravity while the patient is in the semierect position.

The aspirate is submitted for bacteriologic evaluation, which is clinically important in the treatment of renal carbuncle. This condition has recently been successfully treated solely with antibiotics. The usual renal abscess is caused by staphylococci sensitive to penicillin. In one case, a renal carbuncle caused by penicillin resistant Klebsiella bacteria was aspirated and appropriate antibiotic therapy instituted instead of treatment by "trial" (61).

Renal biopsy
Percutaneous biopsy of renal lesions is carried out in a manner similar to cyst aspiration. This requires, however, a specially trained cytologist, since occasionally only scattered tissue fragments are obtained from the small gauge needle used for biopsy. After the lower pole of the kidney is outlined, the depth to this area is measured and the needle inserted toward the lateral portion of the lower pole. The optimal angle for biopsy is determined by the position of the transducer (57).

SOLID TUMOR

The following criteria are used to diagnose a solid neoplasm:

1. The distal wall is irregular in contour.
2. The distal wall is unsharp and has lower level echoes than does the proximal boundary due to small change in acoustic impedance.
3. Poor through transmission, since a large amount of sonic energy is attenuated in passing through the tumor mass.
4. Presence of internal echoes that define the acoustic inhomogeneity of the

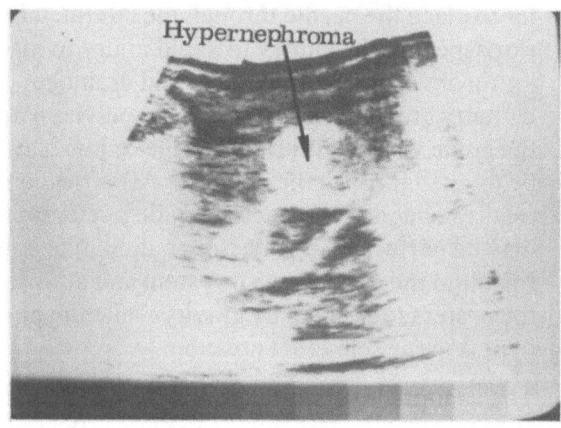

FIGURE 10.11 (a)
Prone longitudinal scan. Space-occupying mass in upper pole. Solid hypernephroma with high through transmission. Head is toward the right.

FIGURE 10.11 (b)
Prone longitudinal scan. Echo-free mass splitting apart lower calyceal echo pattern. Hypernephroma (2 cm) without degeneration. Head is toward the right.

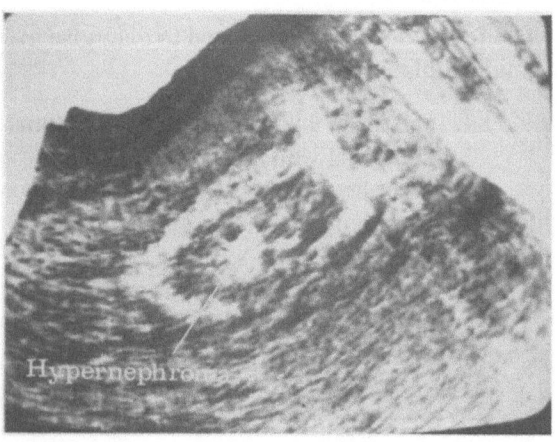

mass. It may be necessary to increase the sensitivity setting to demonstrate internal echoes from an acoustically heterogeneous lesion. The tumor may arise in any portion of the kidney (Fig. 10.11a and b).

DEGENERATING SOLID TUMORS

As a tumor enlarges it outgrows its blood supply, producing fluid-filled necrotic spaces that increase through transmission. At low sensitivity, the anterior and posterior walls may be visualized without the appearance of internal echoes, simulating a cystic structure. At higher gain settings the tumor will fill-in with internal echoes (31) (Fig. 10.11c). If the tumor has a largely necrotic center, an echo-free area will remain at high sensitivity. However, this anechoic region will be smaller than the tumor outlined at low sensitivity.

In conclusion, by varying the sensitivity of the receiver, ultrasound differentiates a fluid-filled cyst from a solid mass with a high degree of accuracy. This method is reliable for differentiating between the two lesions when there is continued sonic homogeneity within the margin of the mass at different gain settings and no change in the sharpness of the margins. Electrical noise and reverberation may cause artifacts on the B-scan in the anterior portion of the cyst. This difficulty can be resolved by using A-mode simultaneously with the B-scan.

RENAL TRANSPLANT

Serial measurements of the size of renal transplants are useful for detecting acute or intermediate rejection and shrinkage secondary to progressive fibrosis of the transplanted kidney. Magnification on x-ray film (approximately 20 percent) should be corrected before the film is compared with the undistorted scan. The transplanted kidney is located in the iliac fossa obliquely. The A-mode or B-scan may be used. More accurate measurements are possible when the A-mode echoes are superimposed on a calibrated scale. Newly devised electronic calipers may also be employed.

Longitudinal and transverse scans are made

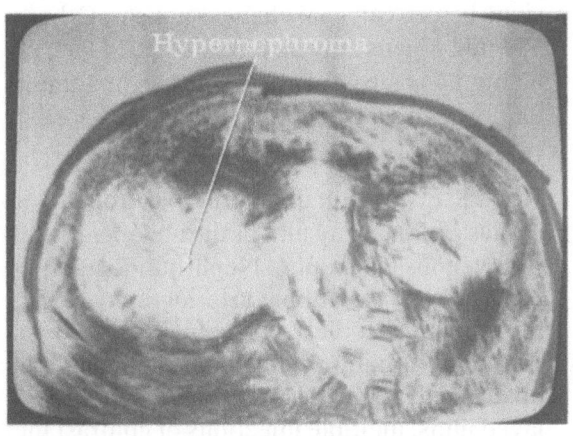

FIGURE 10.11 (c)
Prone transverse scan. Irregular mass in upper pole of kidney. Scattered internal echoes of low amplitude are noted and a high through transmission pattern is observed when compared with the opposite side. Degenerating hypernephroma.

with respect to the lie of the transplanted kidney; length, width, and volume can be calculated. When the kidney becomes edematous, the sonolucency and through transmission are increased compared with the previous sonogram; size and volume are also increased.

Asymptomatic infections often appear since the immune mechanisms of these patients are altered by steroids, cytotoxic drugs, or radiation therapy. The infections are commonly perirenal abscesses at the site of renal transplantation. Scanning may demonstrate collections of serum, lymph, blood, or pus as a sonolucent area that may fill-in with echoes at high sensitivity, depending on the content of the fluid (5,49). Morphologic changes in renal transplants are of diagnostic value. A sudden increase in renal size implies acute rejection. Absence of expected hypertrophy of the transplant after several months suggests chronic rejection and fibrosis. Dilatation of the calyceal system indicates ureteral obstruction (40).

POLYCYSTIC AND MULTICYSTIC DISEASE

Polycystic disease is usually diagnosed by observing bilaterally enlarged renal outlines with a markedly lobulated outer contour, as contrasted to the smoother surface produced by hydronephrosis. In addition, septae in the polycystic kidney have a random distribution, as opposed to the central radiation noted in the obstructed and dilated calyceal system (11) (Fig. 10.12a and b). It is difficult to distinguish a hydronephrotic sac from a massive renal cyst severely compressing the remaining renal parenchyma. Multicystic disease of the newborn cannot be differentiated sonographically from nonfunctioning hydroenphrosis produced by congenital obstruction of the ureteropelvic junction. Ultrasound is an excellent screening procedure for the diagnosis and follow-up of polycystic disease. Early cystic changes will enlarge the kidney but will not distort the calyces sufficiently to be detected on routine intravenous urograms. Gray scale may identify cystic le-

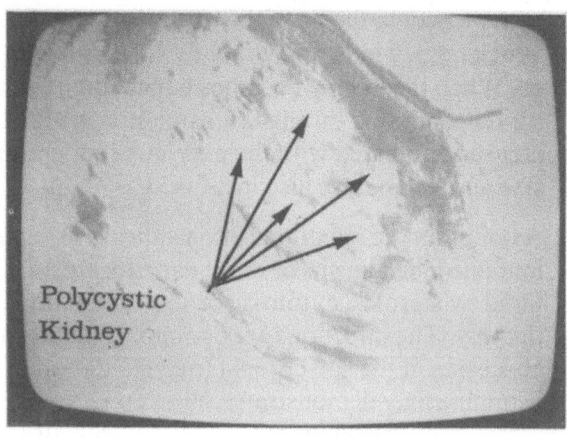

FIGURE 10.12 (a)
Prone longitudinal scan. Enlarged and distorted renal outline. Multiple anechoic regions are noted in a diffuse arrangement. Septations between anechoic cysts are random in distribution. Opposite kidney with similar appearance. Polycystic disease.

FIGURE 10.12 (b)
Prone transverse scan. The enlarged renal outline has sonolucent regions with random septations.

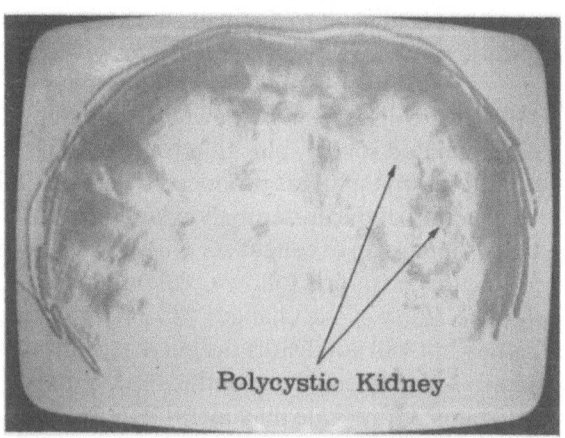

sions before calyceal changes appear. Other affected organs may also be studied. Thus, sonography is ideal for evaluating asymptomatic family members.

OBSTRUCTIVE UROPATHY

Routine evaluation of obstructive uropathy includes a plain x-ray film of the abdomen and intravenous urography. Nephrotomography, retrograde pyelography, arteriography, and renal isotope studies are frequently added for further information. The poor function of the obstructed kidney generally necessitates delayed films, multiple injections of contrast medium, significant radiation exposure, and patient discomfort associated with long waiting periods on a hard table top. The rapid diuresis created by the high osmolality of the contrast medium may increase intrapelvic pressure sufficiently to produce pyelosinus reflux or even peripelvic extravasation of urine and contrast medium into the retroperitoneum (65).

Urinary stasis may have obstructive and nonobstructive mechanisms. Impedance to urine flow commonly occurs with tumors and calculi of the kidneys, ureters, and bladder. Other ureteral problems include anomalies of insertion, stricture, stenosis, and pregnancy. Abnormal ureteral compression is associated with retrocaval ureter, lymphadenopathy, abscess, hematoma, or aberrant vessel. Prostatic hypertrophy and posterior urethral valves produce functional bladder outlet obstruction. Nonobstructive stasis follows neurogenic dysfunction of the bladder, chronic inflammatory conditions, atony of the ureters with high urinary output, and vesicoureteral reflux (35).

The size of the obstructed kidney may appear increased, normal, or decreased. Interstitial edema of acute obstruction tends to enlarge the renal parenchyma. Back pressure atrophy of the cortex associated with chronic obstruction produces a small kidney in most cases (35). Thus, renal size may only be interpreted as a diagnostic aid with reference to sequential studies over a known period of time.

Pathophysiologic changes in the pelvicalyceal system reflect the degree and duration of in-

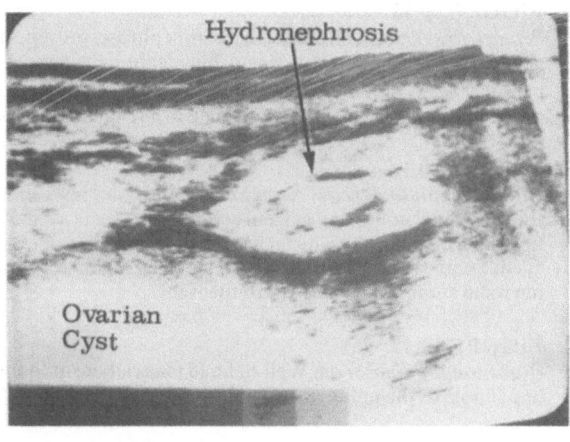

FIGURE 10.13
Prone longitudinal scan. Splitting of the renal sinus echoes forming an avoid echo pattern. Obstructive hydronephrosis.

FIGURE 10.14
Prone longitudinal scan. Moderate hydronephrosis thins the renal parenchyma and produces sacs of fluid with septae radiating centrally.

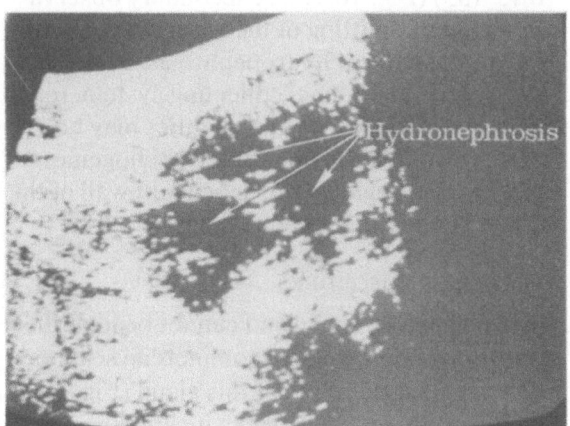

creased pressure and damage from superimposed infection. Dilatation of the calyces, infundibulae, and pelves usually progresses proportionately. However, the extrarenal pelvis acts as an hydraulic buffer, sparing infundibulae and calyces as it dilates to dissipate the increased pressure. Hence, marked pyelectasis with normal infundibulae and calyces in the presence of an extrarenal pelvis can be seen. This sign is of limited value however since the anatomy of the renal pelvis may not be known at the time of study.

Earliest pathologic changes of chronic increased pressure occur in the calyceal system. Blunting of the acute forniceal angle is followed by flattening and eventual clubbing of the calyx. Subtle calyceal alterations often escape ultrasonic detection (25) due to the resolution of the 2.25-MHz transducer routinely used in renal scanning. The renal sinus is the invagination of the renal hilus and contains the renal pelvis, major calyces, and main renal vessels. The principle ultrasonic observation in early obstruction is dilatation of the renal sinus produced by intrarenal enlargement of the renal pelvis and adjacent major calyces.

The first sonographic finding in hydronephrosis is "splitting" of the renal pelvicalyceal echoes (72) (Fig. 10.13). This corresponds to distension of the calyces and infundibulae so that distinct echoes are reflected by each inner wall surrounding the anechoic collected urine. As dilatation proceeds, degeneration of renal tissue distorts the calyces into pockets of urine retained within compressed atrophic bands of renal tissue (Fig. 10.14). This produces the picture of thick septae dividing a large cystic collection, with a shell of remaining sonolucent cortex discernable at medium sensitivity (60). Further destruction of the cortex by back pressure atrophy and infection may result in a lobulated renal periphery, simulating a multilocular cyst (11). Eventually, only a fluid-filled sac of variable size can be visualized (72) (Fig. 10.15). Differentiation between hydronephrosis and pyonephrosis may be suggested by observing irregularity of tissue septae dividing cystic collections within the kidney (60).

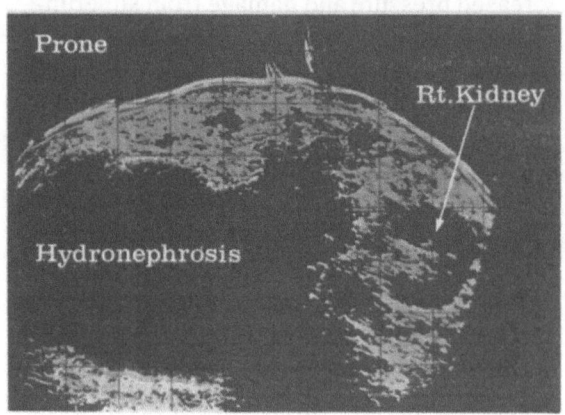

FIGURE 10.15

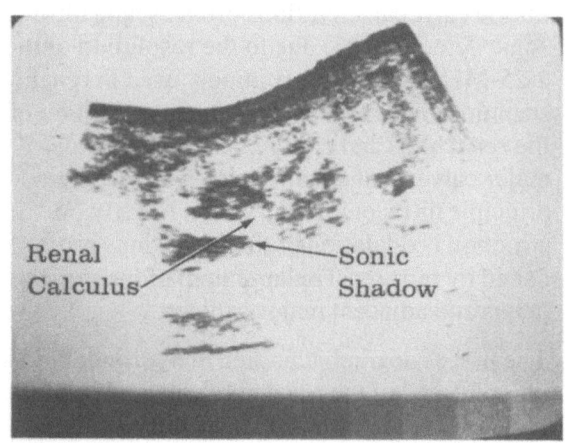

FIGURE 10.16

FIGURE 10.17 (a)

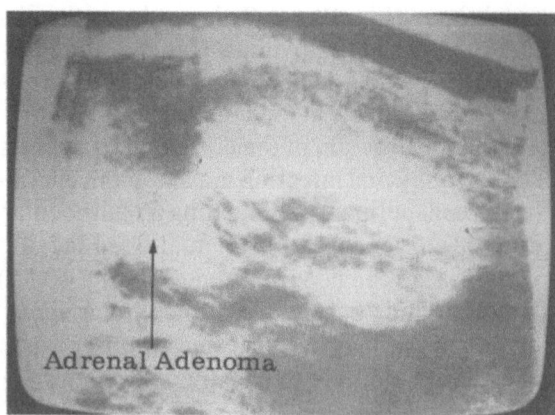

FIGURE 10.15
Prone transverse scan. Massive hydronephrosis presents as an echo-free sac without distinguishing features. No renal parenchyma is noted. This cystic lesion must be differentiated from other cysts by the absence of a renal outline.

FIGURE 10.16
Prone longitudinal scan. A very dark echo complex within the gray renal collecting system echoes represents a calcified renal calculus. The distal wall of the kidney is not imaged. Sonic shadowing may be produced by highly reflecting renal stones. Head is toward the right.

FIGURE 10.17   (a)
Prone longitudinal scan. Well-defined mass adjacent to the upper pole of the kidney. Adrenal adenoma.

Chronic obstructive uropathy is often clinically silent in the adult and frequently presents with vague symptoms in the pediatric age group and geriatric population. Radiation hazard is significant in the former and full cooperation for satisfactory radiologic examination is limited in the latter. Ultrasound may be used in these patients as a simple and atraumatic screening procedure and for routine follow-up studies in high-risk cases.

RENAL CALCULUS

The high calcium content of the usual radiopaque calculus markedly reflects sound waves. The stone will appear as a stronger echo than that from the surrounding calyceal echoes, if it acts as a specular reflector. An irregular or amorphous calculus will act as a diffuse reflector and be difficult to image. The lack of through transmission may cast a "sonic shadow." (33) (Fig. 10.16). A secondary observation may be splitting of the renal sinus echoes due to concurrent hydronephrosis. In the presence of a dilated renal collecting system, renal calculi of lower reflecting qualities may be demonstrated as low-amplitude echogenic masses lying against the dependent wall of the dilated collecting system.

PERIRENAL DISORDERS

The normal adrenal gland cannot be identified with currently available commercial scanners. Cystic or solid tumors of this gland (Fig. 10.17a and b) or areas of heavy calcification may be

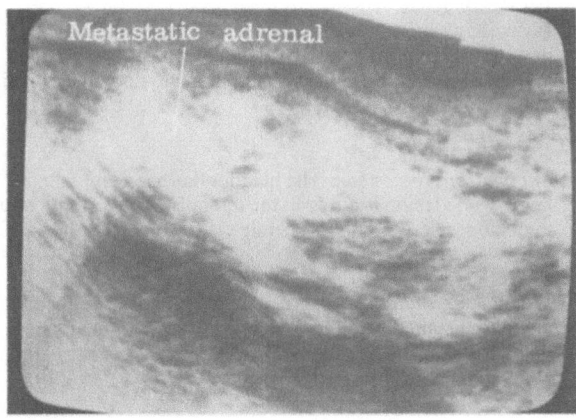

FIGURE 10.17 (b)

FIGURE 10.17 (b)
Prone longitudinal scan. Echo-poor mass of large size with high through transmission. The tumor deforms the upper pole of the kidney and is separated by a echogenic boundary. Typical appearance of metastatic adrenal gland. Bronchogenic carcinoma.

FIGURE 10.18
Prone transverse scan. The ovoid outline of the left kidney is clearly imaged. The right renal outline is not visible and the low level echoes of the hepatic parenchyma fill the region normally reserved for the right kidney. Congenital absence of the right kidney.

FIGURE 10.19
Supine longitudinal scan. The ptotic kidney lies in an extremely caudal position. This pelvic kidney must be differentiated from a displaced kidney due to a mass lesion.

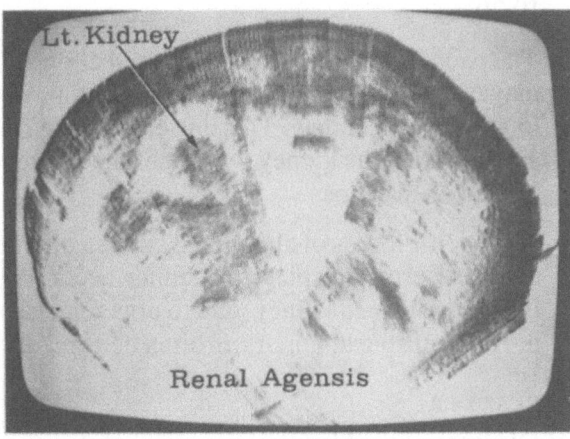

FIGURE 10.18

FIGURE 10.19

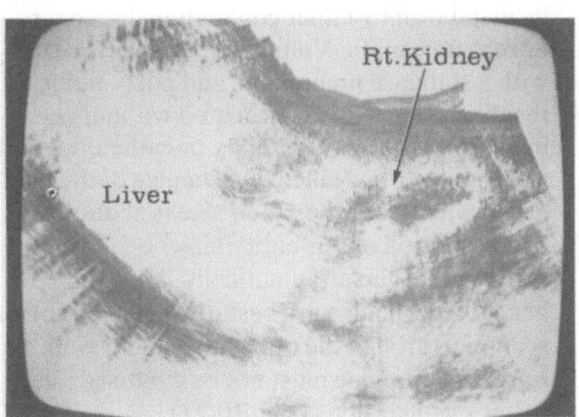

visualized, if they are sufficiently large. Adrenal metastases are common in patients with breast and bronchogenic carcinomas and may be completely asymptomatic. For this reason, these tumors are generally large when discovered (18). The tendency for internal degeneration often causes the metastatic adrenal tumor to simulate a cystic lesion (31). For definitive diagnosis, a line of demarcation between the upper pole of the kidney and the suprarenal mass must be demonstrated.

Perirenal fluid collections may be easily detected. Hematoma secondary to trauma and lymphocele or seroma from regional surgery appear as echo-free regions, often conforming to local fascial planes. Perirenal abscess presents as an irregular echo-free area with scattered internal echoes at higher sensitivity, corresponding to necrotic debris. A search should be made for associated intrarenal changes, such as hydronephrosis (60).

THE DISPLACED KIDNEY

Renal aplasia and ectopia result in the inability to detect the characteristic sonographic appearance of the kidney in the expected retroperitoneal scanning region (Fig. 10.18). Scanning must be performed, with the patient in the supine position, over the lower abdomen to show a pelvic kidney. The ptotic kidney (Fig. 10.19) will change location with vigorous respiration or when the position of the patient

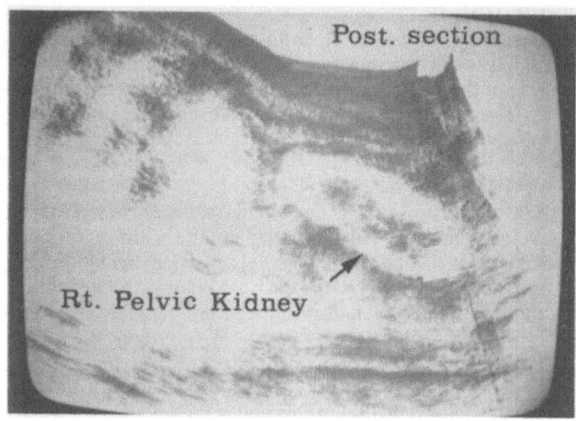

FIGURE 10.20

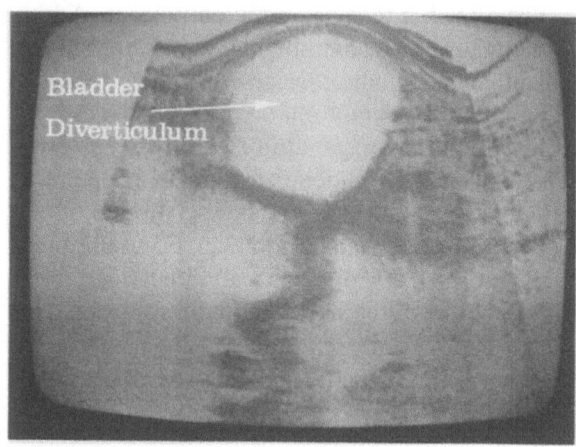

FIGURE 10.21 (a)

FIGURE 10.21 (b)

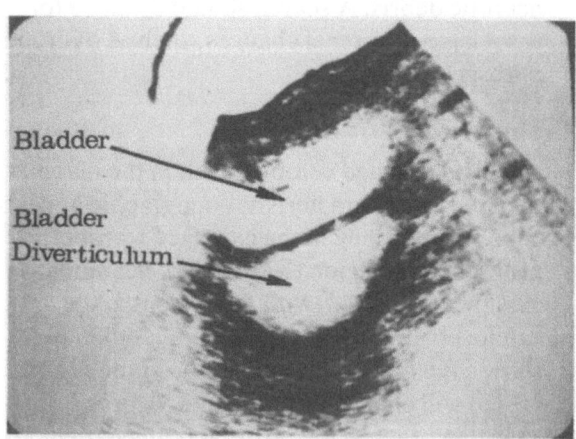

FIGURE 10.20
Erect longitudinal scan. Change in position of a mobile kidney is best demonstrated by scanning in the prone position and then rescanning in the erect position to document maximum renal excursion.

FIGURE 10.21   (a)
Supine transverse scan. The bladder has been emptied. A large cystic lesion is noted in the left pelvis. Diverticulum of the bladder may simulate a pelvic cystic tumor.

FIGURE 10.21   (b)
Supine longitudinal scan. An echo free cystic area occurs distal to the filled bladder. This diverticulum of the bladder is separated from the bladder by the thickness of the bladder wall. Head is toward the right.

changes. The sitting-erect position permits the greatest movement to be documented (Fig. 10.20).

The psoas muscle is ovoid in cross-section and may occasionally simulate the renal outline in longitudinal scanning. This muscle is distinguished from the kidney by the absence of central calyceal echoes.

The vector forces of abdominal and retroperitoneal masses will displace the kidney accordingly. The displaced kidney, due to organomegaly or retroperitoneal tumors, is often deformed.

BLADDER

Diseases of the bladder may manifest themselves in the upper abdomen. This is especially true of bladder outlet obstruction, causing proximal hydronephrosis, and bladder tumors metastatic to aortic lymph nodes.

The fluid-filled bladder is distinctly outlined on its distal wall by either conventional scanners or real-time units. Volume is readily assessed with a standard nomogram, and postvoiding residual urine may be measured without resorting to intravenous urography or catheterization techniques. Fluid-filled diverticulae of the bladder may be seen when their size is about 2 cm. The evolution of this entity may be followed sequentially and atraumatically. Laterally placed diverticulae are best examined by sector scanning through the opposite bladder wall. Large diverticulae must not be confused with pelvic cystic lesions (Fig. 10.21).

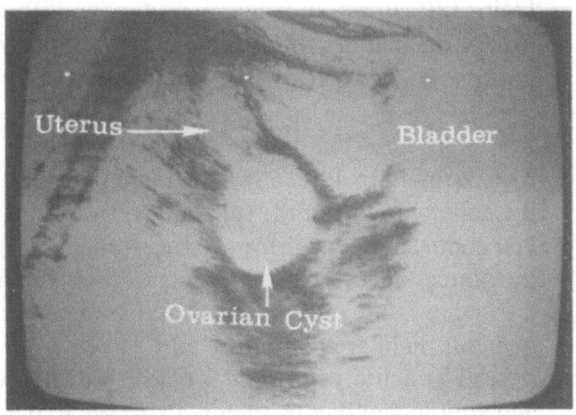

FIGURE 10.22

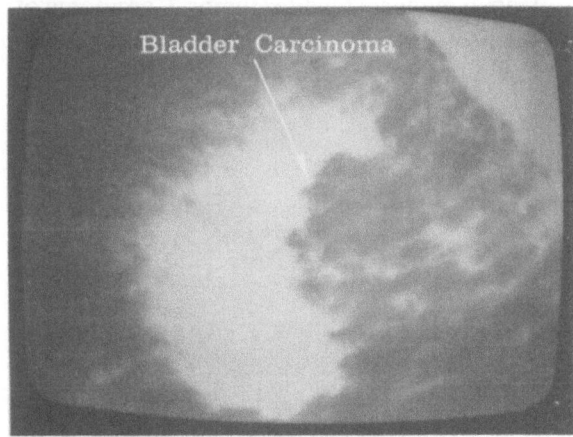

FIGURE 10.23

FIGURE 10.24

The contour of the bladder is studied for symmetry, distensibility, and tumor masses. Extravesical lesions such as uterine fibroids and ovarian cysts (Fig. 10.22) may distort the normal contour of the bladder wall. The expected uniform expansion of the bladder is evaluated by monitoring its shape with increasing urine or fluid volumes. Alterations in distensibility occur with infiltrating carcinoma and chronic inflammatory disease. Masses adherent to the wall of the bladder are most often malignant (Fig. 10.23). However, tumors in the region of the base of the bladder may represent benign prostatic hypertrophy. This glandular enlargement generally appears echogenic (Fig. 10.24). Current resolution does not permit differentiation of submucosal extraluminal lesions from sessile intraluminal tumors.

FIGURE 10.22
Supine longitudinal scan. The distal wall of the bladder is indented by an echo-free ovarian cyst.

FIGURE 10.23
Supine transverse scan. Mucosal bladder tumor is demonstrated on the right bladder wall. This tumor is echogenic. Papillary bladder carcinoma.

FIGURE 10.24
Supine transverse scan. The base of the bladder is pushed anteriorly. A large echogenic mass of sharply outlined tissue appears to be a common appearance of prostatic hypertrophy.

FIGURE 10.25
Supine transverse scan. Echo-poor mass extends through the bladder base. The mass is irregular and not well-encapsulated. Prostatic carcinoma.

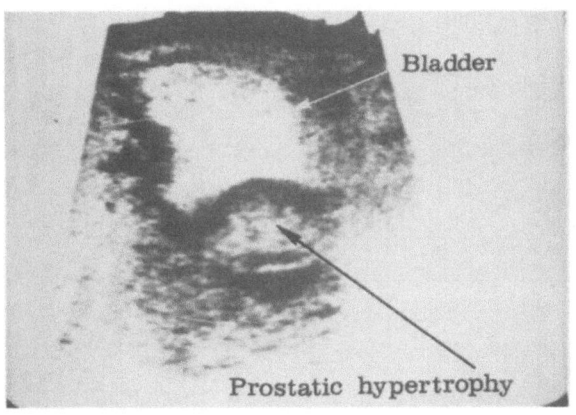

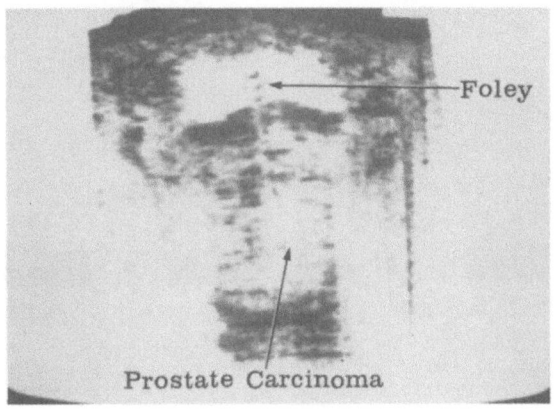

Using ultrasonic guidance, percutaneous puncture of the bladder for diagnostic or therapeutic purposes is performed quickly and simply.

PROSTATE

The normal prostate may be studied through the sonic window of the full bladder or by special endoscanners, with a rotating transducer introduced transrectally or transurethrally. The normal prostate may be visualized as an homogeneous, light gray structure at the bladder base. The acutely inflamed prostate is enlarged and sonolucent due to edema. Prostatic hypertrophy produces an enlarged organ of dark gray echoes. If this enlargement protrudes into the bladder base, it may be difficult to distinguish from a mucosal bladder tumor. Carcinoma of the prostate may appear as an irregular mass of low-amplitude echoes (63) (Fig. 10.25).

bibliography

1. Aoyagi K. History of ultrasound in application from industry to medicine. *Ultrasonics 9*:128–138, 1966.

2. Ballantine HT, Bolt RH, Hueter TF, Ludwig GD. On the detection of intracranial pathology by ultrasound. *Science 112*:525–528, 1950.

3. Ballantine HT, Hueter TF, Nauta WJH, Sara DM. Focal destruction of nervous tissue by focused ultrasound: Biophysical factors influencing its application. *J Med 104*:337–341, 1956.

4. Bartrum RJ. Practical consideration in abdominal ultrasonic scanning. *N Engl J Med 291*:1068–1070, 1974.

5. Ben-ora A. Ultrasound diagnosis of lymphoceles following renal transplantation. *Proceedings of the 20th Annual Meeting of the American Institute of Ultrasound in Medicine*. New York, Plenum Press, in press.

6. Brascho DJ. Diagnostic ultrasound in radiation treatment planning. *J Clin Ultrasound 1*:320–329, 1973.

7. Brown RE, Sartin, M, Bogardus CR. Patient contours in radiation therapy planning. Talk presented at the 17th Annual Meeting of the American Institute of Ultrasound in Medicine, November *16–20, 1972.*

8. Carlsen EN. Gray scale ultrasound. *J Clin Ultrasound 1*:190–195, 1973.

9. Carlsen EN. Ultrasound physics for the physician. A brief review. *J Clin Ultrasound 3*:69–75, 1975.

10. Crafts R. *Human Anatomy*, New York, Ronald Press, 1966.

11. Damascelli B, Lattuada A, Musumeci R. Two dimensional ultrasonic investigations of the urinary tract. *Br J Radiol 41*:837–843, 1968.

12. Doust BD, Maklad NF. Ultrasound B-mode examination of the gall bladder. *Radiology 110*: 643–647, 1974.

13. Dussik KT, Dussik F, Wyt L. Auf dem Wege zur hyperphonographie des Gehirnes. *Wien Med Wschr 97*:425–429, 1947.

14. Eastcott GHH. *Arterial Surgery*. Philadelphia and Toronto, J B Lippincott, 1969, pp. 278–285.

15. Feigenbaum H, Chang S. *Echocardiography*. Washington and Philadelphia, Lea and Febiger, 1972.

16. Filly RA, Freimanis AK. Echographic diagnosis of pancreatic lesions. *Radiology 96*:575–582, 1972.

17. Firestone FA. The supersonic reflectoscope for interior inspection. *Metal Prog 48*:505–512, 1945.

18. Forsyth JR, Gosink BB, Leopold GR. Ultrasound in the evaluation of adrenal metastases. *Proceedings of the 20th Annual Meeting of the American Institute of Ultrasound in Medicine*. New York, Plenum Press, in press.

19. Freimanis AK, Asher WM. Development of diagnostic criteria in echographic study of abdominal lesions. *Am J Roentgenol 108*: 747–755, 1970.

20. Garrett WJ, Robinson DE. *Ultrasound in Clinical Obstetrics*. Springfield, C C Thomas, 1970.

21. Goldberg BB, Goodman GA, Clearfield HR. Evaluation of ascites by ultrasound. *Radiology 96*:15–22, 1970.

22. Goldberg BB, Harris K, Brooker W. Ultrasonic and radiographic cholecystography. *Radiology 111*:405–409, 1974.

23. Goldberg BB. Ultrasound aortography. *JAMA 119*:353–358, 1966.

24. Goldberg BB. *Diagnostic Ultrasound in Clinical Medicine*. New York, Grune & Stratton, 1975.

25. Goldberg BB, Ostrum BJ, Isard HJ. Nephrosonography: ultrasound differentiation of renal masses. *Radiology 90*:1113–1118, 1968.

26. Green WM, King DL, Casarella WJ. Differential diagnosis of echo free renal masses. *Proceedings of the 20th Annual Meeting of the American Institute of Ultrasound in Medicine*. New York, Plenum Press, in press.

27. Greene D, Steinback HL. Ultrasonic diagnosis of Hypernephroma extending into the inferior vena cava. *Radiology 115*:676–680, 1975.

28. Haber K, Asher WM, Freimanis AK. Echographic evaluation of diaphragmatic motion in intra-abdominal diseases. *Radiology 114*: 141–144, 1975.

29. Halpert B, Willms RK. Aneurysms of the aorta. *Arch Pathol 74*:163–168, 1962.

30. Hancke S, Holm HH, Koch, F. Ultrasonically guided percutaneous find needle biopsy of the pancreas. *Surg Gynecol Obstet 140*:361–364, 1975.

31. Hassani N, Bard R, von Micsky LI. Through Transmission patterns in solid tumors. *Proceedings of the 20th Annual Meeting of the American Institute of Ultrasound in Medicine*. New York, Plenum Press, in press.

32. Hassani N. Ultrasonic appearance of pedunculated uterine fibroids and ovarian cysts. *J Natl Med Assoc 66*:432–434, 1974.

33. Hassani N. Sonic shadow sign. *J Natl Med Assoc 67*:307–310, 1975.

34. Hassani N. Method and usage of ultrasound in clinical medicine. *J Natl Med Assoc 67*:41–45, 1974.

35. Hodson, JC, Craven DJ. The radiology of obstructive atrophy of the kidneys. *Clin Radiol 17*: 305–320, 1966.

36. Holm HH, Rasmussen SN, Kristensen JK. Errors and pitfalls in ultrasonic scanning of the abdomen. *Br J Radiol 45*:835–840, 1972.

37. Holm HH. Ultrasonic scanning in the diagnosis of space-occupying lesions of the upper abdomen. *Br J Radiol 44*:24–36, 1971.

38. Holm HH. Ultrasonic diagnosis of arterial aneurysms. *Scand J Thor Cardiovasc Surg 2*: 140–146, 1968.

39. Holmes HH, Rasmussen SN, Kristensen JK. Ultrasonically guided percutaneous puncture technique. *J Clin Ultrasound 1*:27–31, 1973.

40. Holmes JH. Urologic ultrasonography, in King DL (ed): *Ultrasound Diagnosis*. St. Louis, CV Mosby, 1974.

41. Howry DH, Bliss WR. Ultrasound visualization of soft tissue structures of the body. *J Lab Clin Med 40*:579–583, 1952.

42. Jensen FL, Kristensen JK, Holm HH. Long term results of ultrasonically guided percutaneous aspiration of renal cysts. *Proceedings of the 20th Annual Meeting of the American Institute of Ultrasound in Medicine*. New York, Plenum Press, in press.

43. Kahn PC. Pancreatic echography. in Eaton SB, Ferrucci JT (eds): *Radiology of the Pancreas and Duodenum*. Philadelphia, London, and Toronto, WB Saunders, 1973.

44. King DL. Ultrasonography of echinococcal cysts. *J. Clin Ultrasound 1*:286–291, 1973.

45. Kossoff G. Display techniques in ultrasound pulse echo investigation; a review. *J Clin Ultrasound 2*:61–72, 1974.

46. Lande A, Bard R. Arteriographic diagnosis of pedunculated splenic cysts. *Angiology 25*: 617–620, 1974.

47. Langevin MP. Les andes ultrasonares. *Rev Gen Elect 23*:626–634, 1928.

48. Leopold GR, Talner LB. Renal ultrasonography: an updated approach to the diagnosis of renal cyst. *Radiology 109*:671–678, 1973.

49. Leopold GR, Asher WM. Diagnosis of extraorgan retroperitoneal space lesions by B-scan ultrasonography. *Radiology 104*:133–138, 1972.

50. Leopold GR, Asher WM. Deleterious effects of gastrointestinal contrast material on abdominal echography. *Radiology* 98:637–640, 1971.

51. Leopold GR. Pancreatic echography: a new dimension in the diagnosis of pseudocyst. *Radiology 104*:365–369, 1972.

52. Leopold GR. Echographic study of the pancreas. *JAMA 232*:287–289, 1975.

53. Leopold GR. Echographic and radiological documentation of spontaneous rupture of a pancreatic pseudocyst into the duodenum. *Radiology 102*:699–700, 1972.

54. Leopold GR. A review of retroperitoneal ultrasonography. *J Clin Ultrasound 1*:82–87, 1973.

55. Lyon MF, Simpson GM. An investigation into the possible genetic hazards of ultrasound. *Br J Radiol 47*:712–722, 1974.

56. Marich KW, Zatz LM, Green PS, Suarez JR, Macovski A. Real time imaging with a new ultrasonic camera: Part 1. In vitro experimental studies on transmission imaging of biological structures. *J Clin Ultrasound3*:5–16, 1975.

57. Mazzeo CE, Goldberg H. Ultrasonic localization and guidance for renal biopsy. *Proceedings of the 20th Annual Meeting of the American Institute of Ultrasound in Medicine.* New York, Plenum Press, in press.

58. Meyers MA. Distribution of intra-abdominal malignant seeding: dependency on dynamics of flow of ascitic fluid. *Am J Roentgenol 119*: 198–206, 1973.

59. Mountford RA, Wells PNT. Ultrasonic liver scanning; the A-scan in normal and cirrhosis. *Phys Med Biol 17*:261–265, 1972.

60. Mountford RA, Ross FGM, Burwood RJ. The use of ultrasound in the diagnosis of renal disease. *Br J Radiol 44*:733–742, 1971.

61. Pedersen JF, Hancke S, Kristensen JK. Renal carbuncle: antibiotic therapy governed by ultrasonically guided aspiration. *J Urol 109*: 777–778, 1973.

62. Pepper HW, Keene J. Use of Simethicone in abdominal echotomography. *Proceedings of the 20th Annual Meeting of the American Institute of Ultrasound in Medicine.* New York, Plenum Press, in press.

63. Po JB, Sample WF, Marks L, Glenny R. Prostatic scanning with gray scale ultrasound. *Proceedings of the 20th Annual Meeting of the American Institute of Ultrasound in Medicine.* New York, Plenum Press, in press.

64. Porrath S, Avallone LT. Radiation planning using ultrasound. *Proceedings of the 20th Annual Meeting of the American Institute of Ultrasound in Medicine.* New York, Plenum Press, in press.

65. Rabinowitz JG, Keller RJ, Wolf BS. Benign peripelvic extravasation associated with renal colic. *Radiology 86*:220–226, 1966.

66. Rasmussen SN. Liver volume determination by ultrasonic scanning. *Br J Radiol 45*:579–585, 1972.

67. Rasmussen SN. Spleen volume determination by ultrasonic scanning. *Scand J Haematol 10*: 298–304, 1973.

68. Rogoff MS, Lipchick OE. Aneurysms of the abdominal aorta, *in Abrams LH (ed): Angiography.* Boston, Little Brown, 1971, pp. 759–772.

69. Rosch J. *Roentgenology of the Spleen and Pancreas* Springfield, C C Thomas, 1967.

70. Sample WF, Po JB, Gray RK, Cahill PJ. Gray-scale ultrasonography: techniques in pancreatic scanning. *Appl Radiol 10*:63–67, 1975.

71. Sample WF, Po JB, Poe ND, Graham LS, Bennett LR. Correlative studies between multiplane tomographic unclear imaging and gray scale ultrasound in extra and intra-hepatic abnormalities. *Proceedings of the 20th Annual Meeting of the American Institute of Ultrasound in Medicine.* New York, Plenum Press, in press.

72. Sanders RC, Bearman S. B-scan ultrasound in the diagnosis of hydronephrosis. *Radiology 108*: 375–382, 1973.

73. Segal LB. Ultrasound diagnosis of an abdominal aortic aneurysm. *Am J Cardiol 17*:101–103, 1966.

74. Steinberg I, Stein HL. Visualization of abdominal aortic aneurysms. *Am J Roentgenol 95*: 684–695, 1965.

75. Stuber JL, Templeton AW, Bishop K. Sonographic diagnosis of pancreatic lesions. *Am J Roentgenol 116*:406–412, 1972.

76. Takashi K, Morikawa Y. Ultrasonographic determination of the splenic size and its clinical usefulness in various liver diseases. *Radiology 115*:157–161, 1975.

77. Taylor KJW. Gray scale ultraonography in the differential diagnosis of chronic splenomegaly. *Proceedings of the 20th Annual Meeting of the American Institute of Ultrasound in Medicine.* New York, Plenum Press, in press.

78. Taylor KJW, Glees JP, Smith IA, Carpenter DA. Accuracy of gray scale ultrasonic examination of the liver. *Proceedings of the 20th Annual Meeting of the American Institute of Ultrasound in Medicine.* New York, Plenum Press, in press.

79. Taylor KJW, Carpenter DA. The anatomy and pathology of the porta hepatis demonstrated by gray scale ultrasound. *J Clin Ultrasound 3*: 117–119, 1975.

80. von Micsky LI. Clinical sonography in urology. *Urology, 1*:506–522, 1974.

81. von Schreeb T, Arner O, Skovsted G. Renal adenocarcinoma: is there a risk of spreading tumor cells in diagnosis of renal cyst? *Scand J Urol Nephrol 1*:270–276, 1967.

82. Walls WJ, Gonzalez G, Martin NL, Templeton AW. B-scan ultrasound evaluation of the pancreas. *Radiology 114*:127–134, 1975.

83. Weill F, Maurat P. The sign of the vena cava:

Echotomographic illustration of right cardiac insufficiency. *J Clin Ultrasound* 2:27–32, 1974.

84. Weill F, Elsenschar A, Aucent D, Bourgoin A, Gallinet D. Ultrasonic study of venous patterns in the right hypochondrium: an anatomical approach to differential diagnosis of obstructive jaundice. *J Clin Ultrasound* 3:23–38, 1975.

85. Wells PNT. *Physical Principles of Ultrasonic Diagnosis.* London and New York, Academic Press, 1969.

86. Zatz LM, Marich KW, Green PS, Lipton MJ, Suarez JR, Macovski A. Real time imaging with a new ultrasonic camera: Part 2. Preliminary studies in normal adults. *J Clin Ultrasound* 3: 17–22, 1975.

index

A

Abdominal aorta
  anatomy of, 73
  aneurysms in, 72, 75–76, 77
  para-aortic lymphadenopathy in, 76–77
  sonoanatomy of, 73
  sonography of, 72
  sonolaparotomy of, 74
  sonopathology of, 74–77
Abscesses, 99
  hepatic, 37–38
  perirenal, 115
  splenic, 52
  subphrenic, 88
Acoustic impedance, definition of, 4–5
Adrenal gland, tumors of, 101, 114–115
Air, effects on ultrasound transmission, 28, 44, 58
Amebic abscess, hepatic, 37
A-mode (amplitude mode)
  description and use of, 9–10
  simultaneous display of, with B-scan, 27
Ampulla of Vater, carcinoma of, 69
Anechoic disc, 77
Aneurysms, of abdominal aorta, 72, 75–76, 77, 99
Angulation, technique of, 25
Anterior projection, techniques of, 24
Aorta, ultrasonography of, 8
Artifacts, from reverberation, 7, 20, 30, 77
Ascites, ultrasonography of, 8, 38, 69, 88, 89–92, 94
Asthma, 39
Astigmatism, incorporation into focus system, 20
ATC-series, technique of, 24
Attenuation
  definition of, 3–4
  technique of, 26
Axial resolution, description of, 6

B

Barium, effects on ultrasound transmission, 28
Barium titanate, piezoelectric properties of, 2
Beam path, 5
Beam width, definition of, 3
Bile duct
  carcinoma of, 69
  obstruction of, 38
Biliary tree sonopathology of, 45–46
Biopsy
  of kidney, 109
  puncture, ultrasonic guidance,

  of liver, 39–40
  of pancreas, 70–71
Bladder
  cancer of, localization of, 94
  sonopathology of, 116–118
  ultrasonography of, 21
Blood, pools of ultrasonography of, 8
Blood vessels, sonography of, 72–84
B-mode (brightness mode), description and use of, 10
Bone, scanning impedance of, 4, 5, 9, 20, 28
Breast carcinoma
  perirenal metastases of, 115
  radiation planning for, 94
Brucellosis, splenic pathology in, 52
B-scan, simultaneous display of, with B-scan, 27

C

Calculi, renal, 101, 114
Cancer
  of bladder, 116–118
  of gallbladder, 44, 45
  hepatic, 34–36
  of pancreas, 55, 56, 65–69
  of prostate, 118
  renal, 109–110
  in retroperitoneum, 98
  sonolocalization of, 94
Carcinogens, ultrasound and, 21
Cathode ray tube, function of, 13–14
Center control, 20
Cervix, cancer of, localization of, 94
Choledochal cyst, sonopathology of, 45
Cirrhosis, ultrasonic detection of, 38, 39
Colon, ultrasonography of, 24
Contrast, enhancement of, 20
Crystal, size of, beam width and, 16
Cycle, definition of, 2
Cyst(s)
  choledochal, 45
  hepatic, 29, 34, 36–37
  renal, 28, 65, 100, 101, 104, 105–109
  splenic, 50, 51
  ultrasonography of, 8, 27, 28, 42, 48

D

Damp control, 18
Damping system, pulse characteristics and, 16, 17
Decibel, derivation and use of, 3
Decubitus projection, techniques of, 25

Delay control, 18
Depth control, 18
Depth resolution, description of, 6
Diagnostic medicine, wavelengths of sound in, 1
Diaphragm
   anatomy of, 85–86
   sonoanatomy of, 86
   sonography of, 85–88
   sonolaparotomy of, 86–87
   sonopathology of, 87–88
Diffuse reflection, 8
Digital read out, 20
Directivity, of ultrasound, 8
Display modes, description of, 9–13
Dissecting aneurysms, of abdominal aorta, 76, 77
Duodenum, ultrasonography of, 24

E

Ear, highest frequency audible to, 1
Echinococcal splenic cysts, 50
Echo pattern, definition of, 3
Echo shape, 5
Emphysema, 39
   effects on diaphragm, 88
Emphysematous cholecystitis, 44
Envelope detection, 18
Erase switch, 20
Erect projection, technique of, 25

F

Fluid, retroperitoneal, 99
Focusing, of beam, 18
Frequency, definition of, 2
Fusiform aneurysms, of abdominal aorta, 75

G

Gain control, 18
Gain setting, 26
Gallbladder
   acute cholecystitis in, 42, 43–45
   anatomy of, 40–41
   cancer of, 44, 45
   congenital absence of, 43
   gallstones in, 43–44
   sonoanatomy of, 41
   sonolaparotomy of, 41–43
   sonopathology of, 43–45
   ultrasonography of, 20, 23, 40–45
Gallstones, ultrasonic detection of, 43–44
Gas
   in bowel, 60
      effects of, 26
Gastrointestinal tract, radiographic contrast, effects
      of, 26

Gaucher's disease, splenic pathology in, 53, 54
Gel, for ultrasonography, 21
Genetics, ultrasound effects on, 21
Graticule, 20
Gray-scale imaging, description and use of, 10–11

H

Heart failure
   ascites from, 89
   hepatic effects of, 38, 77, 78
   inferior vena cava in, 77, 78
Hematoma perirenal, 115
Hemidiaphragms, sonography of, 86
Hemolytic anemia, 50, 54
Hemorrhage, 99
   intra-abdominal, 88
Hepatitis, ultrasonic detection of, 38
Hepatoma, ultrasonic detection of, 36
Hodgkin's disease
   sonographic studies on, 94
   spleen pathology in, 54
Huygen's principle, 8
Hydatid cysts, ultrasonic detection of, 36–37
Hydronephrosis, sonopathology of, 113, 114
Hypernephroma, ultrasonic detection of, 22

I

Iliac crest, as reference point, 23–24
Inferior vena cava, 77–84
   anatomy of, 78–79
   sonoanatomy of, 79–82
      shifting method for, 80–82
   sonography of, 77–78
   sonopathology of, 82–84
   tumor or thrombus in, 84
Inflammation, hepatic, 37–38
Intensity, of ultrasonic beam, definition of, 3
Intensity control, 18
Intensity modulation, definition of, 10
Intercostal section, technique of, 25

K

Kidney
   anatomy of, 101
   biopsy of, ultrasonic guidance of, 109
   calculi in, 101, 114
   cancer of, 28
      radiation planning for, 94
   cysts in, 28, 65, 100, 101, 105–109
      puncture, 106–109
   displaced, 115–116
   hydronephrosis of, 101
   obstructive disease of, 112–114
   perirenal disorders of, 114–115

polycystic and multicystic disease of, 111–114
pseudotumor of, 49
sonoanatomy of, 101–104
sonolaparotomy of, 104–105
transplants of, 20, 101, 110–111
tumors of, 109–110
ultrasonography of, 22–24, 100–117

L

Lateral resolution, description of, 6, 7
Lead zirconate, piezoelectric properties of, 2
Leiomyomata, ultrasonography of, 27, 28
Left lower quadrant, ultrasonography of, 24
Left upper quadrant, ultrasonography of, 24
Leukemia, spleen pathology in, 51, 52, 54
Linear Transducer Array, 13
Liposarcomas, ultrasonography of, 28
Lithium sulfate, piezoelectric properties of, 2
Liver
    anatomy of, 29–30
    cirrhosis of, 38, 39, 53
    cysts of, 29, 34, 36–37
    enlargement of, 38–39, 77, 84
    guided puncture biopsy of, 39–40
    hepatitis in, 38
    inflammatory processes of, 37–38
    metastases, 34–36, 38, 42
    sonoanatomy of, 30–32
    sonolaparotomy of, 32–33
    sonopathology of, 33–39
    ultrasonography of, 8, 9, 22–24, 27, 29–40
    volume determination of, 39
Longitudinal decubitus, technique of, 25
Lung
    difficulties of scanning through, 9, 26, 94
    tumors of, 88
LXP-series, technique of, 24
Lymph nodes, enlarged, in retroperitoneum, 97–98
Lymphadenopathy, para-aortic, 76–77
Lymphomas, ultrasonography of, 27, 51, 94
Lymphosarcoma, spleen pathology in, 54

M

Magnification, of echoes, 20
Metals, effects on ultrasound transmission, 28
Metastases
    ascites from, 89
    hepatic, 34–36, 42
    pancreatic, 69
    perirenal, 115
Minus sections, 23
M-mode (motion mode), description and use of, 10
Multicystic disease, of kidney, 111–114
Myelofibrosis, 50
    spleen pathology in, 54

O

Octoson, 23

P

Pancreas
    anatomy of, 56
    cancer of, 55, 56, 65–69
    cysts of, 42, 70
    inflammation of, 62–64
    percutaneous fine needle biopsy of, 70–71
    pseudocysts of, 28, 43, 55, 64–66
    sonoanatomy of, 57–60
    sonolaparotomy of, 60–62
    sonopathology of, 62–71
    ultrasonography of, 24
Pancreatitis, ultrasonic detection of, 44
Para-aortic lymphadenopathy, of abdominal aorta, 76–77
Patient
    contour of, in planning radiation therapy, 93–94
    preparation for ultrasonography, 21
Pediatrics, ultrasound use in, 15
Pelvic bone, as scanning impediment, 26, 96
Pelvic kidney, 115
Pelvic organs, ultrasonography of, 21
Pericardial effusions, ultrasonography of, 8
Peristalsis, effect on ultrasonography, 24
Phased Linear Array, 13
Phrenic nerve, paralysis of, 88
Piezoelectric properties, of ultrasound, 1, 2
PLS-series, technique of, 25
Plus cuts, 23
Polaroid picture(s)
    marking of, 27
    visual orientation of, 27
Polycystic disease, of kidney, 111–114
Polycythemia vera, 50
Port margins, delineation of, by sonography, 94
Porta hepatis
    sonolaparotomy of, 33
    sonopathology of, 70
Portal vein, sonoanatomy of, 46
Posterior projection, techniques of, 25
Power switch, 18
Prostate
    cancer of, localization of, 94
    sonopathology of, 117, 118
Pseudocyst, pancreatic, 28
Psoas muscle, ultrasonography of, 24
PTC-series, technique of, 25
Ptotic kidney, 115–116
Pulmonary disease, sonopathology of, 87–88
Pulse characteristics, damping system and, 16, 17

Q

Quartz, piezoelectric properties of, 2

R

Radiation therapy
    organ evaluation in, 94
    sonography use in planning for, 93–94
Real-time scanner, 12
Real-time scanning
    description and use of, 11–13
    systems, 13
Receiver, function of, 13
Recording, of ultrasonographic data, 20
Reflecting interface, distance measurement of, 7–8
Reflection processes, diagram of, 4
Reflectivity, of ultrasound, 8
Reflex cholecystitis, 44
Reject control, 18, 19
Repetition rate, definition of, 6–7
Resolution, definition of, 5–6
Respiration, effects of, 26
Retroperitoneum
    anatomy of, 95–96
    sonoanatomy of, 96
    sonography of, 95–99
    sonolaparotomy of, 96–97
    sonopathology of, 97–99
Reverberation phenomena, description of, 7
Reverse sonic shadow, 28
Ribs, scanning impedance by, 9
Riedel's lobe, 39
Right lower quadrant, ultrasonography of, 24
Right upper quadrant, ultrasonography of, 23–24

S

Sarcoid, splenic pathology in, 52
Scale, 20
Scan, orientation of, 27
Scanning, types of, 22, 23
Sensitivity setting, 26
Sickle cell disease, 50
Signal amplifier, function of, 13
Signal processing, description of, 16–19
Snell's law, 8
Sonoanatomy
    of diaphragm, 86
    of gallbladder, 41
    of kidney, 101–104
    of liver, 30–32
    of pancreas, 57–60
    of retroperitoneum, 96
    of spleen, 48–49

Sonolaparotomy
    by B-mode, 10
    of deep lesions, 94
    of diaphragm, 86–87
    of gallbladder, 41–43
    of kidney, 104–105
    of liver, 32–33
    practical aspects of, 21–23
    of retroperitoneum, 96–97
    of spleen, 49–50
Sonopathology
    of biliary tree, 45–46
    of diaphragm, 87–88
    of gallbladder, 43–45
    of kidney, 105–117
    of liver, 33–39
    of pancreas, 62–71
    of retroperitoneum, 97–99
Sound
    definition of, 1
    wavelengths of, 1
Sound waves
    medium effects on, 3
    properties of, 2–3
Spleen
    anatomy of, 47–48
    anomalies of, 50
    congestion in, 53
    cysts of, 50, 51
    in Gaucher's disease, 53
    hematologic disorders of, 50–51, 52
    inflammation of, 52
    sonoanatomy of, 48–49, 103
    sonolaparotomy of, 49–50
    sonopathology of, 50–54
    trauma to, 51–52
    ultrasonography of, 9, 24, 27, 47–54
    volume determination in, 53–54
Splenic vein, 48, 49, 59
Stomach, ultrasonography of, 24
Subcostal section, technique of, 25
Subpulmonic effusion, 88
Superior mesenteric vein, 59
Supine longitudinal scan, techniques of, 24
Supine transverse scan, 24
Symphysis pubis, as reference point, 23

T

Teratomatous splenic cysts, 50
TGC control, 26
Thoracoabdominal aneurysms, 75
Thrombi
    in abdominal aorta, 76
    of inferior vena cava, 84
Time gain compensation (TGC), 18
Tissue, ultrasonic damage to, 3

Titanates, use in ultrasonography, 2
Topographic marking, of suspicious area, 27
Transducer(s)
   beam patterns of, 14
   body marking with, 27
   components of, 14–15
   contact of, 25–26
   far field of, 15
   focused type, 15
   function of, 13, 15
   mounting of, 15
   near field of, 15
   optimal crystal size of, 15
   positioning of, 22–23
Transmissivity, of ultrasound, 8
Transmitter, function of, 13
Transplants, kidney, *see under* Kidney
Transverse decubitus projection, technique of,
   25
Tuberculosis, splenic pathology in, 52
Tumors. (*See also* Cancer)
   ultrasonography of, 28

U

Ultrasonic waves, nature of, 1
Ultrasonography
   of abdominal aorta, 72–77
   artifacts in, 7, 20
   of blood vessels, 72–84
   of diaphragm, 85–88
   equipment for, 13–20
   factors affecting normal image, 26
   identification by, 23–28
   of inferior vena cava, 77–84
   of liver, 8, 9, 22–24, 27, 29–46
   main system control in, 18–20
   of pancreas, 24, 55–71
   patient preparation for, 21
   physician's role in, 22
   principles of, 1–28
   reference points of, 23
   of retroperitoneum, 95–99
   of spleen, 47–54
   technologist in, duties of, 21–22
   topographic marking in, 27
Ultrasound
   biophysical effects of, 20–21
   genetic effects of, 21
Umbilicus, lead marker for, 23
Uterus, cancer of, radiation therapy planning in,
   94

V

Vascular anatomy, of pancreatic region, 61–62
Velocity, definition of, 2

Video display, 18
Video signal, 18

W

Wavelength, definition of, 2

X

Xiphoid process (of sternum), as reference point, 23